Psychoanalytic Approaches to Addiction

CURRENT ISSUES IN PSYCHOANALYTIC PRACTICE
Monographs of the Society for Psychoanalytic Training

CURRENT ISSUES IN PSYCHOANALYTIC PRACTICE

Monographs of the Society for Psychoanalytic Training
Number 3

Psychoanalytic Approaches to Addiction

Edited by

Angelo Smaldino, Ph.D.

BRUNNER/MAZEL, PUBLISHERS • NEW YORK

Library of Congress Cataloging-in-Publication Data
Psychoanalytic approaches to addiction / edited by Angelo Smaldino.
     p.   cm. — (Current issues in psychoanalytic practice : no. 3)
   Includes bibliographical references.
   ISBN 0-87630-644-X
     1. Compulsive behavior—Treatment.   2. Psychoanalysis.
   I. Smaldino, Angelo.   II. Series: Current issues in psychoanalytic
   practice (Brunner/Mazel Publishers) ; no. 3
     [DNLM: 1. Compulsive Behavior—therapy.   2. Psychoanalytic
   Therapy.   3. Substance Dependence—therapy.   W1 CU788LD no. 3 / /
   WM 176 P9733]
   RC533.P74   1991
   616.85'20651—dc20
   DNLM/DLC
   for Library of Congress   91-357
                                                                        CIP

Published by
BRUNNER/MAZEL, INC.
19 Union Square
New York, NY 10003

Manufactured in the United States of America

10   9   8   7   6   5   4   3   2

Contents

Foreword

The Editorial Board of *Current Issues in Psychoanalytic Practice* is pleased to sponsor this monograph on addictions. Dr. Angelo Smaldino, Guest Editor of this volume, has assembled an excellent group of clinicians who have laboriously worked with addicts of all types for many years. These clinicians may be regarded as pioneers, in that most psychoanalysts, until very recently, have shunned the addictive personality, contending that he or she was not amenable to psychoanalytic therapy.

One of the many lessons we learn from the pages of this monograph is that it is a trying, tedious, and tumultuous ordeal for both therapist and patient to help the latter move toward gratifying him- or herself in live interpersonal relationships, rather than depend on any of the addictions noted in the papers presented herein.

The addictive personality is frequently a very infantile personality. Consequently, he or she provokes many strong countertransference reactions. As we note, the patient under discussion can induce in the therapist rage, helplessness, depression, and withdrawal. Of course, these are the emotional states of many addicts who, in their unique way, are trying to find a partner to help them cope with their maladaptive lifestyle.

Whether we work with addictive personalities or not, the articles in this monograph will help us understand better the dynamics of many seriously disturbed patients and also assist us in dealing with their chaotic transference reactions, acting out, and difficult resistances with more finesse.

HERBERT S. STREAN, D.S.W.
Editor

vii

Contributors

Joshua F. Cohen, M.S.   Psychotherapist in private practice in Evanston, Illinois; Director, the Summer Doctoral Program of the Institute for Clinical Social Work; Past Director, Community Mental Health Program of the University of Chicago; taught at Chicago Institute for Psychoanalysis and the Illinois School for Professional Psychology; trained at the Columbia University School of Social Work, the Chicago Institute for Psychoanalysis, and the Committee on Human Development of the University of Chicago.

Arthur S. Liebeskind, M.D.   Chief Psychiatrist/Medical Director, Lower East Side Service Center, a multi-modal agency specializing in the treatment of substance abusers in New York City; in private practice of psychoanalytically oriented psychotherapy; graduated from Downstate Medical School; psychiatric residency at Bronx Municipal Hospital and Bellevue; former Clinical Associate in Psychiatry at New York Medical College and an attending at Metropolitan Hospital at the substance abuse service.

Eleanor Bartholomae Liebowitz, Ph.D.   Senior member and faculty member at the New York Center for Psychoanalytic Training; member and training analyst, the National Psychological Association for Psychoanalysis; in private practice on Long Island, New York.

Mitchell May, M.S.W.   Board of Directors, faculty, training and supervising analyst, Training Committee, New York Center for Psychoanalytic Training; Clinical Director, Addictions Unit, Center for Creative Living; Board of Directors, Senior Member, Society for Psychoanalytic Training; private practice, New York City.

Elaine V. Siegel, Ph.D.   Senior analyst of the Society for Psychoanalytic training; in private practice on Long Island; for 14 years, Director of the motor development unit at Suffolk Child Development Center, a research unit of the State University of New York, Stony Brook; author of 20 articles and two books.

Angelo Smaldino, Ph.D., C.S.W., J.D.   Psychoanalyst in private practice in New York City and in Port Washington, Long Island; senior member, training and control analyst, New York Center for Psychoanalytic Training and the National Psychological Association for Psychoanalysis; faculty and Dean of Training, New York Center for Psychoanalytic Training.

Carol Smaldino, M.S.W.   Private practice, Port Washington, New York; Supervisor, New Hope Guild; author of papers on countertransference dynamics; presently writing a book on the art of setting limits for children and parents.

Psychoanalytic Approaches to Addiction

Observations on Countertransference, Addiction, and Treatability

Mitchell May, M.S.W.

It has been observed that when individuals enter psychoanalytic treatment, it is not always clear what has brought them to the analyst. The same is true of anyone seeking treatment who is preoccupied with the use of alcohol and/or drugs. When a patient says at the beginning of treatment, "I'm in an unhappy love relationship," do we tell this patient, "Go. Give up the relationship. Then the analysis can begin"? No, we listen and start exploring the patient's love life. And as we begin to understand and share our observations with the patient, we hope the patient will begin to observe his/her own contribution to his/her own script of life. Does the patient who suffers from a relationship with a substance deserve any less in our treatment? If we don't say, "Give up this relationship," to the first patient, what would prompt us to say it to the second? Yet many people in the mental health professions say just that, "Go. Give up the drug. Then I will treat you."

As we know, countertransference reactions can impede analytic work, and sometimes they can stop the work before it starts. This paper will examine certain types of transference and countertransference reactions in working with a patient who uses a substance such as alcohol or drugs.

1

Transference and Countertransference

Relationships have unconscious wishes attached to them, which are used for defense and are need gratifying; often they serve the repetition compulsion. The relationship between a patient and a substance has all of these ingredients attached to it. There is a transference to the substance. It may be a relationship with a nonperson, but it is a relationship just the same. By developing an in-depth understanding of the derivatives attached to the unconscious transference to the substance and of the uniquely characteristic way the patient handles the preoccupation, and by being able to sit with the pain and anxiety of the patient who continues with his/her addiction (transference) to the substance, the analyst may give the patient a sense of acceptance. Sending the patient to be detoxed before beginning treatment separates the patient from the symptom before the patient is ready to separate. More importantly, the prospective patient may feel rejected because a part of him- or herself, the substance use, is in fact being rejected. The rejection could impede analytic work needed to help the patient develop a transference to the analyst through the analytic process. The transference to the substance could shift to the analyst, which could then begin a new identification, and develop a shift from a punitive to a more benign superego.

Sitting with the patient and his/her continued transference to the substance could cause frustration, anxiety, and possibly anger in the analyst. Yet, by developing the ability to sit with the patient, the analyst will in time be able to help the patient give up the substance. If medical assistance is needed, seeking such help can then be viewed as part of the patient's wish to change, not unlike any other change coming out of analytic work.

The ability to tolerate the reactions of any patient is not an easy task. The development of tolerance and acceptance of all our patients' reactions depends on our own feelings, thoughts, and fantasies about our patients. When these feelings are unconscious, they can impede the work of the analysis and are viewed as countertransference reactions. When they become conscious, they can become manageable. They can be useful for more in-depth understanding of ourselves and, at times, of our patients. As Freud (1910) states,

> We have become aware of the "countertransference" which arises
> in him [the analyst] as a result of the patient's influence on his

unconscious feelings, and we are inclined to insist that he shall recognize this countertransference in himself and overcome it. (pp. 144–145)

Mr. S entered treatment eight years ago because he was experiencing, as he said, "problems with my wife. I sometimes hit my wife." In the initial consultation, he stated very matter-of-factly that he was a consistent cocaine user. He glossed over this fact. For nearly the next two years, the patient talked about his life in a passionless, abstract way as if none of his relationships nor his work situation touched him in any way. Interpretations and explorations of his life were reacted to matter-of-factly as well. Of course, in many ways, this could become frustrating and produce anger in the analyst. At times I wondered what kept this man coming in to see me. He did not seem to have much interest in his marriage, which brought him in to see me in the first place.

Whenever something was expressed that might produce some anxiety, he would begin associating to his cocaine use. In this way, I began to understand his relationship with the drug. It was everything to him. He discussed the adventures he would have buying it, the fantasies he had while high, how he became sexually powerful in his mind, while in reality he felt quite passive and impotent with women. When associating to his use of cocaine, the patient showed some passion. Just talking about cocaine seemed to bring him to life.

As treatment continued, the patient started to become abusive and hostile. He berated my office, my clothes, and me personally. The more he talked about his cocaine use and the fantasies attached to it, the more abusive he became. It is important to note that he seemed to feel that the fantasies were realities. Even though they were inside his mind, they seemed to sustain him through those times when he wasn't high.

There were times when I nearly lost my analytic stance. I was becoming increasingly angry with the constant barrage of insults. When asked why he had to be so abusive, he responded that he was not aware of being insulting, that this was the way he talked to everyone, that people seemed to have no significance for him. I then asked why, if people had no significance for him, he needed to be so abusive? He had no answer and said he really didn't care to pursue it.

As time passed, his abuse of me increased and so did my anger and frustration. At one point, quite angry with this type of degradation, I started to interpret to him that he was trying to defeat me. As with earlier interpretations, for example, of his wish to destroy the analysis and others, this one went absolutely nowhere.

After being in analysis for nearly two years and just before I was to leave on my vacation, he said he thought maybe I was angry with him. This was the first time he had expressed a direct thought about me. Up to this point, whenever he was asked about his feelings toward me, he responded in a manner indicating that I was not really there. This was the beginning of a shift in the transference from the drug to me.

In the months that followed, the patient expressed the wish to give up the drug and began working through his repetition compulsion to use the drug to feel more potent. In the working through process, the inner meanings of his transference to the drug started to become more conscious for him, for example, his passive homosexual stance and conflict, his tremendous rage at everyone for feeling so impotent, and his wish to be taken care of.

He stated, "My cocaine takes care of me better than my mother did." He was then able to explore his anger toward his father for leaving him at an early age. The working through process is still continuing and has deepened since the patient gave up drug use. He now states that during the first two years of treatment, he never really heard what I said, but he remembers that I was always there for him.

The hostility of this patient was a positive sign. It signaled a beginning consciousness of the intimacy developing in the analysis. It signified the fear of that intimacy based on deep-seated distrust, which the analyst must be able to tolerate with a sense of hope that it will lead to the shift from a nonhuman to a human relationship. In order to weather this storm, the analyst must be able, first and most importantly, to tolerate being ignored and, secondly, to tolerate the patient's hostility and the analyst's own hostility.

Cocaine use is a substitute for a human relationship, a transference. The psychoanalytic method is the treatment of choice because our work revolves around working through and resolving infantile transferences. The more we understand, through the psychoanalytic method, about the transference to the substance, the better we are able to help the patient resolve infantile transferences, just as we would with any patient.

Clinical Social Bias

What would make an analyst turn away a prospective patient until the patient had given up the symptom (drug/alcohol)? It could be because the therapist has not recognized this countertransference in him- or herself and overcome it. One of the major contributors to the difficulty for the analyst in working with the substance-using population is social bias.

> Drug abuse is clearly a social, legal and political term with strong derogatory, judgmental explicitness (not just connotations). (Wurmser, 1978, p. 5)

Using such terms as "alcoholic," "drug addict," and "substance abuser" attaches a negative label to the behavior. It is calling the patient a symptom and not a human being. It is labeling a person by his/her behavior and not by his/her total character. This labeling encourages the patient to deny that he/she is a human being with psychological/physiological problems and to see him/herself as a "drug addict" for whom the world should feel sorry. The terms feed a masochistic element in the patient. For the professional, the terms tend to rob the patient of humanness and to develop countertransference problems in the therapeutic attitude.

Because of social biases, anxiety can be experienced, which may lead the analyst to tell the patient to rid him/herself of the substance before beginning analysis. Patients in this population have also been termed "difficult patients," "acting-out patients," "suicidal patients," or "self-destructive patients." These terms can develop a countertransference attitude even before treatment begins. Consider how many patients are hard to reach or "difficult" and possibly even suicidal, yet we do not approach them with the same punitive bias.

Fenichel (1945), among others, has stated that addiction can be a defense against psychosis. At times, it is. But when a patient reveals the drug use, some analysts may, because of their fear of addiction and possible psychosis, make some ill-timed intervention such as psychiatric consultation or detoxification.

Some analysts send the patient for detoxification before treatment. In the detoxification process, the patient can be diagnosed as having, for example, a bi-polar disorder and be placed on a psychopharmaceutical. The pharmaceutical interferes with analytic treatment. In terms

of societal biases, the patient has now been switched to a more acceptable addiction.

Swings between omnipotence and desperation are strong char-
acteristics of the manic-depressive. There are some differences between
the manic-depressive and the patient with a substance problem. The
ego of the manic-depressive has at its disposal the mania and the depressive reactions to alleviate anxiety. The ego of the substance-using patient
feels frustration as pain and does not have full use of mania and depression. The ego of this patient utilizes the substance as a defense. Without
the substance, the patient is left with an ego that suffers.

> The ego of the drug addict is weak and has not the strength to
> bear the pain of depression and easily resorts to manic mecha-
> nisms, but the manic reaction can only be achieved with the help
> of drugs because some ego strength is necessary for the pro-
> duction of mania. (Rosenfeld, 1960, p. 129)

While the manic and the addict are characterized by their eagerness
to avoid—that is, their impotence to tolerate—the impending frustration, the depressed person is characterized by his impotence to
tolerate experienced frustration. Many people become addicts in order
to avoid depression and many addicts become depressed when their
addiction is frustrated. (Federn, 1953, pp. 276–277)

Treatment Issues

Many patients in the substance-using population seem to experience omnipotence of thought, magical thinking, and depression. What
human being does not? The only difference among us is of degree and
intensity. What roles do magical thinking and depression play in the
initial transference? Many patients come into treatment after going
through detoxification at a hospital or rehabilitation center. Consciously,
they feel they have separated themselves from the substance. They
may come into treatment with feelings of euphoria, certain that they
have licked their transference to the substance and are now ready to
pick up the pieces and forge ahead. The analyst can then be "sucked
into" the position of the patient and join the patient in the euphoria.
Many analysts mistake this euphoria for a positive transference. In fact,
the euphoria covers a deep sense of deprivation and desperation. The
omnipotence and magical thinking feed the euphoria. Unconsciously,
there is often still a strong wish for the substance.

Eventually, the underlying feelings will begin to break through, and a deep feeling of deprivation will follow. Then the patient will turn to his/her characteristic way of handling the deprivation and frustration. A patient uses the addiction as a way of trying to stabilize him/herself and to mask the fear of confronting his/her human feelings. The use of the substance is an attempt at self-healing, which ultimately fails.

Though destructive in its effect, drug use might represent an attempt to cope with difficult states. (Rado, 1933)

The analyst who has joined with the patient in euphoria now experiences his/her own negative feelings with regard to the patient's shift. These may include anxiety, depression, and anger.

Other patients enter treatment already experiencing depression. They may have had numerous failed attempts at giving up the substance. Some of the massive denial has been broken. The euphoria of starting afresh has waned and lost some of its defensive purpose. These patients often feel suicidal. The rage about their lives may be manifested by resentments and hostility turned outward sadistically or turned inward masochistically.

Whether the patient is euphoric, depressed, or a combination of these feelings, the analyst could develop a number of countertransferences that could endanger the analytic stance. The analyst may fear the patient's anger, as in the case of a patient who feels resentful, or may experience the fantasy to save the patient who feels sorry for him/herself. A patient with a predisposition for acting on his/her feelings without thinking, at times with drastic results, could induce anxiety, which, in turn, could induce an unconscious wish in the analyst to control the patient. The analyst could concentrate too intently on the reality of the patient's life, making suggestions or telling the patient what to do. This would impede being able to stay with the emotional experiences of the patient. Our own sense of helplessness and hopelessness can become more acute during the crisis situations of the patient. In order to defend our own helplessness, the wish to control the patient could be strengthened.

If we can tolerate our own sense of helplessness as it is stirred up by the patient's attempt at avoiding helplessness, we will have a much greater chance of learning more about it and of communicating different patterns of adaption. (Smaldino, 1983)

We are trying to help the patient tolerate some of his/her over-whelming feelings. In turn, we have to be able to tolerate our own and not act upon them.

Treatment Crisis

As the frustration builds in the analysis, the ego of our patient starts to feel this frustration as pain. The first treatment crisis could emerge. Most patients go through some treatment crisis and want to leave treatment.

> If prepared for the crisis, the therapist will subordinate all his or her efforts in the early stages to preparing for it. Only after the crisis has passed can a deep relationship be established. (Fine, 1982, p. 139)

The treatment crisis is one of the most crucial points of the analysis. It is at this time that the opportunity arises for the analyst to explore the derivatives of the wish to leave treatment. When the crisis arrives, the patient generally reacts to it in his/her own unique way. A patient may miss sessions, refuse to pay the fee, or argue with the analyst. The negative transference develops. With this population, reaction to the treatment crisis is characteristically to go on a substance "binge" unless the treatment crisis has been worked through. It may not involve just missing a session or arguing with the analyst. The patient may disappear for weeks and then wish to return and start again. If the patient returns, we could clarify the inner meaning of the binge, the need to disappear, and the feelings and thoughts of the patient toward the analyst.

In my experience, an understanding of the binge comes from constantly monitoring my own feelings of resentment and anger when the patient disappears—my anxiety about possible suicide, guilt about possible mistakes made, and feelings attached to the patient's action. The binge has been felt as a blow to my narcissism. It is essential to realize from the beginning of analysis that strong and deep feelings will be evoked in us by substance-using patients.

All of these countertransferences can occur regardless of whether the patient has identified the substance problem at the beginning of treatment. A patient may bring up his/her drug use in associations after being in treatment for a time. Revelation of this "secret" can induce anxiety in the analyst.

Keeping secrets from the therapist provokes countertransference
reactions in the practitioner. However, if such reactions are
subjected to self-analysis, they can be used in understanding the
client's conflicts. (Strean, 1985, p. 188)

Some patients develop a crisis situation in order to let the analyst
know about the problem of drug use. Ms. A, a successful professional
woman of 25, displayed a high level of anxiety from the beginning of
her analysis. Her anxiety centered on talking about herself and being
alone with me. This, in turn, brought about associations regarding her
family history. For the first two years of analysis, she came to sessions
regularly and paid her fee. Then she began to be late for sessions and
to miss sessions completely. For a number of months, we explored her
need to be late or to miss sessions. The crisis was developing. I began
to develop feelings of anger, resentment, and frustration related to her
resistances. By analyzing my feelings, I was able to see how my own
frustrations were blocking my ability to observe that these were the
patient's actions and that they might signify a wish on her part to
castrate me and destroy the analysis. At that point, I was free to explore
these issues with the patient and validate my conjecture.

During this period, the patient continued to pay monthly for all
of her sessions. Following my vacation, I reminded her that she had
not paid for the month prior to this, and she indicated she would pay
for the two months at the same time. After some exploration, it became
clear she was having some financial problems, which she did not define.
When I asked if she had any feelings about my absence on vacation, it
became clear that she had missed me, and that, in turn, brought up
feelings of needing another person, something she had never wanted
to feel. To recognize that she needed anyone made her more anxious.
Her dependency wishes were starting to become conscious. The
following month, the matter of paying her fee came up again. I informed
her that we could not continue the analysis unless she was willing to
pay the fee. I told her that we could then continue to analyze her financial
situation and her feelings about paying me.

In the sessions that followed, the patient came in and, with a great
deal of anxiety, told me she had been using cocaine for the past few
months and that the cost of the drug had created her financial dilemma.
The history of her drug use began to unfold, along with the wish to
stop using drugs. She revealed that she had used drugs in the past to
defend against feeling either anxious or dependent on anyone. Sub-

sequently, she paid the fee and continued the analysis. Her drug use was attached symbolically to her father, with whom she had first taken drugs when she was 15 years old. This was part of her transference to the drug, which was shifting and developing into a deeper transference neurosis in the analysis.

Substance-using patients vacillate between positive and negative affective states. During the positive periods, there may be many insights and superficial changes; during the negative, bouts of depression and use of a substance. As I become more familiar with my own bouts of guilt when the patient feels depressed and desperate and with my feelings of grandiosity when the patient seems to be making headway, I am better able to maintain an analytic stance and assist the patient in understanding his/her inner conflicts, forbidden wishes, and punitive superego that underlie his/her symptomology.

Summary

By consistently maintaining an analytic stance, the analyst can sit "equidistant from id, the ego, and the superego" (A. Freud, 1936, p. 28). In this way, we can learn much about the dilemmas of our patients. Schafer, in *The Analytic Attitude,* writes about not responding in kind to the patient's emotional overtures.

> By not responding in kind I mean, for example, not meeting love with love or rejection or exploitation, nor meeting anger with retaliation or self-justification or appeasement and not meeting confidence with thanks or with self-revelation of one's own. (Schafer, 1983, p. 9)

Transference to a substance may mean many different things unconsciously to different patients. It may be a defense against psychosis, an acting out of unconscious wishes and fantasies, a compromise formation, and/or a curative fantasy, as examples.

The use of a substance is a behavior of the patient. It is also a defense used by the ego of the patient. It is essential to become friendly with the defenses of any patient. We need to know what unconscious feeling the patient is trying to ward off and why the patient feels the need to defend at this particular time.

In my work with patients who come to see me with a substance problem, I have learned that a wide range of emotional responses may or may not be verbalized by the patient. Patients who have a transference to a substance are no different from any other human being. We all have, deep inside, feelings of sexuality, aggression, desperation, terror, anxiety, guilt, frustration, and, at times, a sense of helplessness and hopelessness. Patients are often unaware of these deep-seated feelings and cover them with hostility, manipulative behavior, acting out, binges, panic, tremendous denial, and avoidance of dealing with what brought them into treatment in the first place.

If we tend to disregard our anxiety as a signal and clue to the feelings being evoked in us, either by the patient or by our own genetic history, we could become flooded by the patient's desperation, seduced by the patient's quick willingness to give up a substance, frightened by the patient's hostility, and angered by the manipulations and acting out behaviors, which, in turn, can develop a sense of hopelessness in ourselves.

> I would argue that the proper use of countertransference leads to continual self-analysis on the part of the analyst of the most effective kind because it forces the subject (the analyst this time) to face the most painful and embarrassing transferences, even if he does not share this information with anyone. This self-analysis not only takes the sting out of difficulties experienced in the course of doing an analysis but allows the enhancement of the pleasure of being an analyst by the very same mechanism that helps the patient, namely the reduction of the severity of the superego. (Fine, 1985, p. 7)

If we do not deny or avoid the anxiety induced in us, we can become more aware of our own deeper feelings. Instead of feeling frustrated by the substance use of our patients, we can use our bodies and minds as instruments for understanding the deeper, more intense emotions of the patients and can, thereby, assist in the patient's recovery.

References

Federn, E. (1953). *Ego psychology and the psychoses.* New London, CT: Maresfield Reprints.

Fenichel, O. (1945). *The psychoanalytic theory of neurosis.* New York: W. W. Norton.

Fine, R. (1982). *The healing of the mind.* New York: Free Press.

Fine, R. (1985). Countertransference and the pleasures of being an analyst. *Current Issues in Psychoanalytic Practice, 2*(3/4), 3–19.

Freud, A. (1936). *The ego and the mechanism of defense.* New York: International Universities Press, 1966.

Freud, S. (1910). The future prospects of psychoanalytic therapy. *Standard Edition, 11,* 139–152. London: Hogarth Press.

Rado, S. (1933). The psychoanalysis of pharmacotymia (drug addiction). *Psychoanalytic Quarterly, 2,* 1–23.

Rosenfeld, H. (1960). *On drug addiction, psychotic states, a psychoanalytical approach.* London: Hogarth Press.

Schafer, R. (1983). *The analytic attitude.* New York: Basic Books.

Strean, H. (1985). *Resolving resistances in psychotherapy.* New York: John Wiley and Sons.

Smaldino, A. (1983). From action to reflection: New depths in psychotherapy with drug addicts. *Clinical Social Work Journal, 2*(2), 151–163.

Wurmser, L. (1978). *The hidden dimension: Psychodynamics in compulsive drug use.* New York: Jason Aronson.

But I Must Have You in My Life: Thoughts About the Addictive Quality of Some Object Relationships

Elaine V. Siegel, Ph.D.

Toward the end of some lengthy, relatively successful analyses, I was struck by the tenacity with which these particular patients stuck to unsatisfactory, even destructive, relationships. At first glance, object constancy and altruism seemed highly developed in these patients, but as we delved more deeply into the recesses of their psyches, we discovered formidable, in some instances unresolvable, resistances to change in the area of object relationships. Analysis of masochistic tendencies and rescue fantasies proved to be fruitful insofar as the patients were able to gain insight into the origins of their behaviors and were able to make use of their analytic gains in their professional lives. However, nothing changed in the relationships to the people who gave them so much pain. They were, indeed, addicted to the unsatisfactory, often painful interactions that appeared to be the major focus of their inner lives.

Interestingly enough, they were able to describe in detail the effects these relationships had on them, but they rarely, if ever, depicted their important others as people. For the most part, they were content to describe only those actions of their objects that directly impinged on themselves. For the most part, they did so with a singular lack of emotion. Because the surface of their relationships were smooth, these

13

patients were regarded as highly successful by their peers, were even envied for the unswerving devotion they showered upon their mates.

While it was clear from the start that I was in the presence of extraordinarily strong compulsions to repeat, it became more and more difficult to ascertain exactly what was being repeated. Exploration and interpretation of masochistic and sadistic tendencies were simply not applied to their "loved ones" by these patients. They were addicted to them. Slowly, they also became addicted to the analysis, but not the analyst. Summer vacations were experienced as painful loss of nurturance, and occasional inclement weather that made roads impassable was regarded as a personal insult inflicted by fate. The patients claimed to feel panic when there were no sessions. But transference interpretations were received with puzzlement and warded off as irrelevant. Therapeutic stalemates ensued but were resolved when it became clear that these patients were reproducing approximations of their unsatisfactory interactions with ungiving, withdrawn, or coldly domineering mothers.

While this in itself is not a surprising event in any analysis, these patients found it particularly hard to penetrate their need to repeat because they had very early on found a way to soothe themselves and thus to "overlook" and deny the injuries inflicted on them by others. For all of them, masturbation had become the most convenient form of satisfaction to stave off agitation, depression, and pain. Indeed, at times it seemed as though the pleasure in masturbation, discovered late in treatment but very early in life, had skewed their perception of reality. Masturbatory activity was simply not discussed in the beginning and middle phases of these treatments. Its very occurrence at any time was denied until memories and reconstructions finally poured into the transference and allowed these patients to acknowledge actual and symbolic masturbation.

As early as 1897, Freud, in a letter to Fliess, stated that masturbation is the one major habit, the "primary addiction," and it is only as a substitute and replacement for it that other addictions to alcohol, morphine, tobacco, and the like come into existence (Freud, 1985, p. 287). In 1898, he added,

> Left to himself, the masturbator is accustomed, whenever something happens that depresses him, to return to this convenient form of satisfaction. (p. 275)

What was not recognized and known then was that masturbation, besides fulfilling drive needs, can serve as an important defense and can aid in attempted mastery of cumulative trauma. By cumulative trauma, I mean the pervasive impingement on development by an indifferent or hostile environment (Khan & Masud, 1963). Specifically, I refer to the failure of the caretaking person in infancy to provide a protective shield. When this protection does not exist or is withdrawn, the infant has no way to eliminate overwhelming stimuli, and thus a nucleus of pathogenic reactions to the primary caretaker is set up (Spitz, 1965). Most often in these cases, the breakdown of healthy adaptive behavior is between mother and child and becomes visible only in retrospect as disturbance.

What I am postulating for my patients is that normal, age-appropriate masturbation became an adaptation to inadequate or intrusive mothering and was resorted to in an addictive fashion in order to master psychic tension, frustration, and pain. But because of the high degree of pleasure in this self-soothing activity, my patients failed to recognize and then to resolve their object relational conflicts. In adult life, they needed unresponsive, withdrawn, at best neutral, objects in order to retain their solitary pleasure. But their self-soothing activity also served the function of protecting them from the pain of knowing that their "loved ones" were not loving at all.

Having lived for so long in emotional isolation, analytic neutrality was not at all recognized as such, but was interpreted by them as the normal course of events. Thus, in the beginning of treatment, these people seemed to be "good" patients. They talked freely, having always assumed that they must bear the bulk of any human interaction. Contrarily, in the midphases of their analysis, when some resistances had been worked through, my emotional and interpretive presence was felt to be threatening and sometimes overwhelming. In emotionally responding to me, actual and symbolic fantasies of autoerotic self-sufficiency were shaken.

Except for the emptiness and frustration experienced with their mates and lovers, these patients' lives were quite successful. They themselves idealized their own behavior toward spouses and lovers as protective and necessary to their own stability. They were shocked and deeply distressed to discover the consequences of their own addictive behavior. Some clinical examples will illustrate what I mean.

I

Mrs. T, an executive in a major company, presented herself for analysis when she discovered that her husband of three years had taken an insurance policy of $100,000,000 on her life, had failed to enter her name as the coowner of their house, and was no longer sexually interested in her. He did not contribute to household expenses but continually upbraided Mrs. T for "being spendthrift and scatterbrained." Mrs. T described herself as nervous and depressed. She could hardly lie still on the couch. She squirmed and fidgeted as though expecting attack. She reported feeling panicked when, on top of everything else, her husband had discontinued one of her unwanted magazine subscriptions by reporting her dead. Although she did not believe that he wanted to kill her, she felt she could not disregard all the accumulating "evidence." Simultaneously, she had a fantasy of being a heroine in a romantic novel, married to an unfeeling brute, but loved by a charming, though faithless, sailor. This fantasy had its roots in reality. Mrs. T as an adolescent had been in love with a young man who was "socially superior" to her. Her parents were very religious and discouraged her hopes of marrying this young man, claiming that he would seduce and then leave her. Mrs. T believed her parents and with much anguish gave up her suitor. He consequently became a merchant seaman.

Mrs. T stayed celibate until she was 32, when it dawned on her that she would become an "old maid" if she didn't "hurry up." She had been dating Mr. T, a deacon of her church. He quickly acquiesced when she, quite out of character, took the initiative and proposed to him. Their sex life was unsatisfactory from the start. Mrs. T blamed herself for her husband's premature ejaculation and was shocked to discover him masturbating in the shower. She felt rejected but continued to try to please him until she found what she thought was evidence that he wanted to do away with her.

The analysis soon progressed. Mrs. T received promotions, became more sociable, and was able to confront her husband to demand explanations for his behavior. But their relationship remained empty and sexually unsatisfactory. Mr. T declared that he did not want any children, another blow to Mrs. T, which, however, she glossed over. Instead, she began to speak of how quiet and calm her life with Mr. T was in contrast to life with her parents, how he helped her around the house, often brought her presents, and took her on expensive vacations. In all, the former potential murderer was now viewed as a kind protector, of whom she was scarcely worthy.

There remained only two areas of her life she was dissatisfied with: Sex continued to be frustrating and her mother appeared to be jealous of her financial success. Mrs. T's parents disapproved of the ostentation they thought their daughter preferred and badgered her for money and attention. It now became clear that the parents had for a long time used Mrs. T to discharge their own tensions. They both liked to drink in the afternoon and evening ever since she could remember. When she was a teenager, they called Mrs. T into their darkened room and subjected her to "constructive criticism." She was told all about her misdeeds, mainly infractions of the house rules, and was warned that she would come to a bad end. Both parents impressed upon her how they had struggled and sacrificed for her and that she owed them not only obedience but monetary rewards. The Bible was frequently cited. Mrs. T was not allowed to defend herself or to explain her behavior, but was expected to receive all admonitions and rebukes in humble silence. When she cried, she was taunted as a crybaby and as weak.

She recalled with some consternation that she had learned to block out her parents' harangues by silently counting one-two, one-two, over and over again and by staring at her own feet. She claimed that she was counting her feet. As a matter of fact, to this day, she compulsively and frequently counted many things and paired them up. If she were to allow herself to count to three, "a crisis would threaten." These crises consisted of fantasies of being attacked by vicious dogs, of being robbed of all her possessions, of being deserted. Mrs. T was very ashamed of these fantasies and became distraught when she could no longer control them by counting. She suddenly wanted to lash out at her parents and husband and became horrorstruck when she felt a need to attack and beat her nieces and nephews. She reacted in every way as though she had committed all these acts. During this time it was impossible for her to hear and to take in interpretations. She wailed about her "bad character" and counted even more desperately than before.

In the midst of her attempts to control the onslaught of her unleashed identifications with the aggressors in her life, she had a screen memory (Greenson, 1958). She recalled that as a child of three or four, her mother had dressed her in a ruffled sunsuit. Playing in the sand, she forgot to go to the toilet and wet herself. Crying, she went to look for her mother, who was entertaining some neighbors. Mother made fun of her and sent her back out "to dry off the same way she got wet." Sobbing, the little girl found some leaves and tried to dry her pants with them. In this process, she discovered a nice feeling between her legs. With paroxysms of shame and self-disgust, Mrs. T, on the couch, recalled how she had taken off her sunsuit and inserted some leaves in her labia. Other memories of examining her genitals and that of friends followed. Now Mrs. T was convinced that "she had been perverse even as a child," no wonder her parents and her husband thought her inadequate. It was good, in her opinion, that she had them around to guide her.

Very slowly, she began to understand how the good feeling between her legs—she refused to acknowledge the words vagina and clitoris—had helped her to cope with early castration anxiety (Roiphe & Galenson, 1981) and with the threatened loss of her mother's love. More memories of secret doings emerged. When Mrs. T played with her dolls, she spanked them, scolded them, and then pressed them between her legs. At that time, her mother went to work and left the child with her grandparents. Grandpa was enormously interested in the little girl. He liked to see her on the pottyseat Grandma insisted on her using. Grandma disapproved of his interest and yelled at him to chase him away when the little girl attended to her bodily functions. Grandma went so far as to lock her granddaughter into a room while she went to church so Grandpa wouldn't get too close.

While recalling these scenes, Mrs. T could hardly contain herself. She counted even during the sessions to counteract her mounting excitement. Frequent trips to the toilet became necessary during sessions. An anal itch became unbearable. Queried about her body feelings, Mrs. T finally acknowledged infantile seduction at the hands of Grandpa. He had frequently "played with" her by putting his hand on her crotch and tickling her behind. First in the front, then in the back. Sometimes he inserted his finger into her anus. These games went on until Mrs. T was about seven years old. She never told anyone about them because she didn't want Grandpa to stop loving her. He was the only one who was always nice to her!

Then, she contracted impetigo. Mother blamed the grandparents, quit her job, and took over the task of caring for her child again. Under a doctor's instructions, she daily bathed the open sores, reducing the child to screaming fits because of the pain involved. Neighbors intervened and a more humane cure was instituted. Mrs. T characterized this time as "awful. I never took my hand from between my legs when I could help it, but Mom didn't like it and hit me, so I stopped."

Mrs. T clearly had made a link between the guilty doings with her grandfather and the cruel treatment for impetigo. Dreams and association led her to talk about the punishment she was receiving from God and from her mother. Of course, this punishment was perceived as entirely just because she had not even tried to stop the games with grandfather but, rather, had enjoyed them. She carried this equation with her into adult life, apparently in dutiful pursuit of a blameless life, while secretly and obsessively soothing herself first with actual masturbation, then with her ritual counting. This masturbatory equivalent both sustained her and isolated her from meaningful interpersonal contact.

Her analysis did not progress further until she was able to understand and to integrate the function of her "primary addiction."

II

Alexandra came to analysis at the insistence of her parents. They had discovered her homosexual liaison with an older woman. The addictive quality of homosexual behavior has been noted by Socarides (1978) and others. But Alexandra's love affair had an even more obsessive, yet exclusive, dimension of its own. She showed no interest in anyone but Teresita and spent herself in pursuit of this single, elusive person. Teresita was a runner of some fame and a gym teacher. She had become a mother "by consensus," as Alexandra called it. This meant that Teresita had approached a male friend who agreed to impregnate her without making any claims on the child. Alexandra admired this arrangement as definitive proof of Teresita's independence and moral courage as a liberated woman.

Session after session was spent in breathless accounting of Teresita's excellence and her responses to Alexandra. Still, because the focus was always on what Teresita did and on explanations about why she had a right to ward off and to manipulate Alexandra, no picture of her as a person emerged. At first, I could not even ascertain if Alexandra and Teresita had actually met or just talked on the phone at any given point, if they had agreed on a rendezvous or not. Alexandra simply did not answer questions but continued to reflect constantly on her beloved's actions or nonactions vis-à-vis herself. Eventually, it became clear that Alexandra was the only active one. Teresita was in the midst of a painful separation from a long-time female lover who had helped her to raise her daughter. Alexandra eagerly offered herself as a substitute and refused to accept repeated rebuffs.

Not only did the contents of the session prove to be difficult to deal with due to Alexandra's inability to observe herself at first, but it was also difficult to maintain the analytic frame (Langs, 1976). Alexandra's mother called often and refused to accept my nonreporting stance. Although Alexandra was in her late twenties, her mother could not believe that her parenting tasks at this point included staying out of the treatment. She insisted on giving "valuable information" to me by telling me that Alexandra had been the happiest and best adjusted of her many children, tuned in to the needs of her surroundings, and "without a minute of trouble to anyone" until her teen years when she suddenly withdrew and became moody. Alexandra's mother did not seem to hear me when I tried to explain that I could not include her in the analysis, that this was something Alexandra had to do on her own. Mother simply continued talking with the same frenzied quality as her daughter and leaving many messages on my answering machine.

Meanwhile, Alexandra defended her mother's intrusiveness as tenaciously as Teresita's lack of responsiveness.

Alexandra was a poet with a growing reputation. She read her poetry in student centers and to women's groups. She earned little money, taking occasional jobs here and there when she overspent the liberal allowance from her wealthy parents. She passionately defended any and all minority causes, particularly women's rights. Her rather engaging, intense personality always gained her access to the "leading body" of any given group, but this usually came to naught. Each promising political alliance or publishing connection dried up after a short time. Alexandra vigorously denied that her behavior could have anything to do with her many failures.

After about two years, Alexandra made the, to her, startling discovery that her analyst was the only steady and predictable presence in her life. She now experienced my insistence that she make up missed sessions as comforting. This had been a sore point before because her poetry readings frequently took her out of town, as did the fact that her beloved Teresita had moved to Washington, DC. Alexandra might not have money for food or her rent, but she always found ways and means to phone Teresita daily and to spend weekends with her. She had also agreed to contribute a small sum to her analytic fee and used this to berate me for being a money-hungry capitalist. The bulk of the fee was taken care of by her parents.

Sometimes Teresita permitted Alexandra to stay in her apartment, sometimes not. To me, it seemed that Teresita allowed Alexandra to stay when she needed a babysitter. Alexandra agreed, but thought this charming and eagerly involved herself with Teresita's child, who soon clung to her, looking forward to her many visits. During this time, Alexandra's appearance, always somewhat Bohemian, began to be slovenly. She gained weight and could no longer write. She did not meet some of her professional engagements, and showed up at her sessions wild-eyed and obsessed by thoughts of Teresita in another woman's arms.

Little by little we began to make some headway. Alexandra understood that she was acting toward Teresita as her own mother had acted toward herself. For instance, she remembered that her mother had regularly monitored all her childhood friends as to "suitability," showed up at school at various intervals to fight with her teachers about her grades, and had successfully obtained a part in a high school play for her by donating funds for a lavish production. On festive occasions, such as Valentine's Day, she received roses from her mother. This fact was something Alexandra could question. All other intrusions had been rationalized as the right of a concerned mother. Now, Alexandra thought it "extreme" to be courted by her mother and began to chafe under the restrictions still placed on her. Her mother expected Alexandra to check in at least once a week to report where she planned to go and what she had done. It now became clear why the regularity of analytic sessions had appeared as such a burden. It was viewed as a repetition of mother's restrictions.

When Alexandra visited Teresita, she regularly called her own answering machine to make sure that her mother hadn't called her that day. Alexandra also remembered that her mother had often come to sleep in her bed when her father and mother had a fight. The little girl was elected to be her mother's companion when her father was out of town. She was mother's "escort" to weddings, concerts, and the theater. Alexandra reported being at first bored but then highly stimulated by all the attention she gained as the only child in many adult gatherings.

As she began to see more and more parallels between her mother's treatment of herself and her own behavior with Teresita, she had the following dream: She found a dead infant under a tree in the backyard of her childhood home. Shocked, she tried to resuscitate it, without success. Teresita came along and stroked the child, who started to come to life. But Teresita didn't look like herself, she looked like the analyst. Alexandra "couldn't believe that she liked the analyst that much," and she recognized herself in the dead infant.

Now, for the first time she was able to speak about the many lonely hours she spent masturbating compulsively. Analysis of the concomitant fantasies allowed her to recognize the defensive and adaptive qualities of masturbation, including the transferential wish to have sex with her analyst. Masturbation shored up her damaged sense of self. It allowed her to have secrets from her all-powerful mother. Alexandra felt victorious and independent when she masturbated. Soon after this phase, Alexandra began to be more introspective. She characterized her new, calmer mode of interacting with the world and particularly with me as "the real me standing up." At this point she was also able to give up the relentless pursuit of the unresponsive Teresita.

III

Dr. A wanted analysis "because investigation of my inner self is consistent with all I believe." A highly regarded professor at a university, he was fascinated by the application of various investigative tools, among them psychoanalysis, to social, behavioral, and historical phenomena. Cost had prevented him from seeking analysis until a deep depression and a failing marriage drove him to seek help. Nevertheless, it was almost impossible for him to admit that anything was amiss. He spent many of his sessions discoursing brilliantly on the woes of the world or on his latest research. Every now and then he let it slip that he and his wife had not had sexual intercourse for months, that they had agreed to separate financial arrangements, and that a torrid extramarital affair prior to entering analysis had been frightening. He brought in painstakingly detailed computer printouts of his dreams and was disappointed when I thanked him for his thoughtfulness but nevertheless strongly suggested that it would be more fruitful for the analysis to forego some details in favor of spontaneously capturing affective and associative qualities.

He very much wanted to be a good patient but continuously bogged himself down by pursuing with academic punctiliousness many items such as my office decor, which seemed to him to reveal too much of my personal tastes. He eventually became reassured when he saw a picture of Freud's collection in his office at Berggasse 19. It then dawned on Dr. A that I had not defended my choice, merely asked him what it made him think of. He thereafter approved of my technique and declared himself satisfied with his choice of analyst.

But he was less satisfied with my equally neutral stance about his love affair. He wanted to be punished for it. He now claimed to loathe the woman who, he insisted, had liberated his sexuality after many barren years with his wife. But it turned out that his mistress juggled three men simultaneously and had once indulged in homosexual adventures. She also asked him to divorce his wife before he was ready to do so. He berated himself for having misread her so completely.

It soon became apparent that he "misread" his wife as well. He had met her when he was a poor graduate student and she was still an undergraduate. According to him, she had pursued and then seduced him into marriage. A veteran of the disastrous Vietnam War, he smarted under his country's political decisions and saw them as a personal defeat when he met his wife, Jane. She offered temporary solace and a certain amount of "middle class normalcy," which he craved. He insisted that he did not love her even then but had married her to "save himself." Asked from what, he was startled and declared me to be "brilliantly insightful." It had not occurred to him that sleepless nights, difficulties in focusing on tasks, and lack of sexual interest could constitute signs of depression.

Now the analysis moved into a phase in which the intellectually gifted, highly verbal Dr. A discovered that he had no words to describe his feeling states. He actually could not differentiate various emotions. After this discovery, Dr. A's discourse shifted to descriptions of anxiety when Jane demanded to know of his whereabouts down to the last minute, although he had long ago given up his mistress. He consciously felt sadness when Jane refused to let his father's dog into the house and anger when she had no time to cook for him. He took pleasure in feeling himself come alive, but was totally bewildered by the recognition that Jane did not share it. Used to an unresponsive, isolated husband, she was puzzled by his childlike amazement at the wealth of feelings he was experiencing. Jane suspected he had taken another mistress. She angrily withdrew from him, and he plunged back into depression. Simultaneously, a female colleague was promoted. Now Dr. A was convinced that "the world belonged to women." His fantasies became inhabited by Blakeian female monsters, all intent on castrating him in one form or another.

During this difficult time when intellectualization, his major defense, no longer protected him, many childhood memories emerged. His mother, a fragile, depressed woman in chronic mourning for her own mother, had been unable to nurture him. Dr. A's father, a dashing adventurer, had "rescued" the mournful young woman from a rigid, though prosperous, household. His early promises of success fizzled out, and the young couple found itself in financial distress at the birth of their oldest child, Dr. A. A succession of children followed, with the family barely able to survive financially. Dr. A's grandfather provided some funds and became the major source of influence on his oldest grandson. The little boy was precocious intellectually, eager to learn, and obedient. He learned not to expect anything from his mother, but to soothe her and to acquiesce to anything she wanted. Not that she demanded much. Forced by circumstances to go to work without being prepared for it, her scant energies went toward providing food and shelter for her brood. Fights and recriminations between the parents were frequent. Dr. A remembered trying to block out the shouting by humming to himself.

When he was six or seven, he had to wear an eye patch to correct an astigmatism. His teacher in the small midwestern town where they lived declared him incompetent in their reading lessons and ostracized him for holding back the other children. The dismayed child began to doubt the judgment of his family, who thought him intellectually superior. He stopped applying himself in school and failed dismally. But this time his mother came to his rescue. She taught him to read, and his learning capacity once more flourished. Puberty was an agony for him. He detested his bodily changes and decided he was the ugliest boy in the world.

By this time, his father had found a job on the continent. The family moved and the boy found himself stranded in an alien world where the other boys made fun of his American haircut and jeans. His only way of surviving in isolation was to demonstrate intellectual superiority. Just as he was conquering a niche for himself in the foreign school, his father once again failed, and the family returned to the USA. There was no money at all, some of the children were ill, and the father decided to leave for Australia to seek his fortune. Nobody had any time or energy to pay attention to the boy.

Without apparent reason, as he put it, he tried to commit suicide by opening his veins. Later in the analysis, it was possible to reconstruct that he was acting out his mother's suicidal impulse. "She used me as her wailing wall," he said. Consciously, he felt he should be able to help her and that when he couldn't, he was not worthy of living. He was sent to a public mental health clinic where the therapist told him to "stop it."

Always an obedient person, he did stop it—namely, feeling anything at all. He started to live exclusively by, with, and through his intellect. Obviously, this led him to misperceive many situations, especially interpersonal ones. Words and their qualities became his prime focus. He soothed himself by reciting poetry when he couldn't sleep, or by uttering sounds. His computer received the loving attention usually reserved for family and friends. He more and more despised his body, trying to control every aspect of it by diet and exercise.

The question of why he and his wife slept in the same bed yet rarely had sexual intercourse disturbed him, but he could find no answer to the riddle. First, he claimed he needed her because of her superior earning capacity, then, because he felt guilty about betraying her. "But I need her" became a steady refrain in the analysis. In each session, he tried to demonstrate to me that he was only half a human being without her or that he could "not negotiate life without her." He suffered excruciatingly because he was also aware that the relationship hardly deserved that name.

Eventually Dr. A revealed a complicated fantasy of a "love affair with death." He felt "thrilled" by the thought of his own death and in secret masturbated with the thought of how and when his demise would occur. The game plan included his wife's discovery of his body. He quickly chastised himself for this fantasy, mentioning that the thought of inflicting such horror on Jane actually helped to keep him from suicide.

Following the conscious decision *not* to commit suicide, Dr. A made some cautious demands on his wife, advising her that psychoanalytic therapy might be indicated for her as well. Full of hauteur, she informed him that, in contrast to him, she "knew who she was" and refused to accommodate this request. Puzzled by his own unaccustomed anger, he disagreed with her and was doubly puzzled when this disagreement felt "good and right" to him. Instead of castigating himself further, he experienced an upsurge of creative thought, wrote several papers that were well received by his peers, and casually let it drop during sessions that he might be able to get along without Jane. She, on the other hand, did not know how to cope with a husband who was no longer acquiescent and distant. She asked for a divorce. Thrown into a panic, Dr. A fell back on verbal masturbation. In the sessions, he recited poetry and seemed thrilled by the sound of his own voice. These recitations, sometimes in a foreign language, rarely had any but the most casual connection with some banal detail of his life. It was not the contents but the sound of his voice that excited Dr. A.

It has become clear that masochistic submission had become the central masturbatory and addictive focus of his marital life, repeating the inadequate, yet stimulating, relationship with his mother.

Discussion

Three very divergent clinical cases demonstrate the addictiveness of certain early types of object relationships. While each of these patients showed very different character structures and ego strengths, their important interpersonal relationships were addictive and often self-destructive. They simply could not let go of their inappropriate mates and lovers, because these relationships provided the backdrops against which they could play out their autoerotic addiction. This addiction, in itself, proved to be a defense against and adaptation to early relationships with mothers who had failed to provide the average expectable environment (Hartmann, 1939).

Although the patients discussed here had the capacity to invest drive energy in a specific object, seemed able to maintain an emotional attachment despite frustrations, and could even tolerate ambivalence, namely, appeared to have reached the level of object constancy (Burgner & Edgcombe, 1972), they could not love at all. The overwhelming need to repeat the deprivations they had suffered at the need-gratifying level of development (Kris, 1950) pushed them into addictive, dependent, and clinging behavior. They feared the loss of their objects as they feared the loss of their selves, and soothed themselves by masturbation in an effort to save themselves from feeling nothing at all and psychologic emptiness. Inadequate nurturing in early life had forced these patients to use autoerotic adaptations (and defenses) in order to stave off acknowledgement of the partial connectedness to themselves of their important others.

References

Burgner, H., & Edgcombe, R. (1972). Some problems in the conceptualization of early object relationships. *Psychoanalytic Study of the Child, 27,* 283–333. New York: Quadrangle Books.

Freud, S. (1898). Sexuality in the etiology of neuroses. *Standard Edition, 3,* 261–286.

Freud, S. (1985). *The complete letters of Sigmund Freud to Wilhelm Fliess, 1887–1904* (J. M. Masson, ed.). Cambridge, MA: Belknap Press.

Greenson, R. (1958). On screen defenses, screen hunger and screen identity. *Journal of the American Psychoanalytic Association, 6,* 242–262.

Hartmann, H. (1939). *Ego psychology and the problem of adaptation.* New York: International Universities Press.

Khan, M. M. R. (1963). The concept of cumulative trauma. *Psychoanalytic Study of the Child, 18,* 286–306. New York: International Universities Press.

Kris, E. (1950). Notes on the development and some current problems of psychoanalytic child psychology. *Psychoanalytic Study of the Child, 5,* 24–46. New York: International Universities Press.

Langs, R. (1976). *The bipersonal field.* New York: Jason Aronson.

Roiphe, H., & Galenson, E. (1981). *Infantile origins of sexual identity.* New York: International Universities Press.

Socarides, C. W. (1978). *Homosexuality.* New York: Jason Aronson.

Spitz, R. (1965). *The first year of life.* New York: International Universities Press.

Substance Abuse Nightmares and the Combat Veteran with PTSD: A Focus on the Mourning Process

Angelo Smaldino, Ph.D.

There is a special population of substance abusers—men who, in addition to having a severe drug and alcohol problem, also served in combat units during the Vietnam war and were later diagnosed as suffering from PTSD. Though Post-Traumatic Stress Disorder (PTSD), as a diagnosis, is not limited to the combat veteran, its inclusion in the 1980 DSM-III certainly added more dignity and clarity to the complex symptomatology of a significant segment of the Vietnam veteran combat population. Vietnam veterans affected by PTSD suffer from debilitating anxiety, severe depression, sleep disturbance, frightening flashbacks, emotional numbing, sudden and explosive rage reactions, and persistent sense of survivors' guilt, along with problems with drugs and alcohol.

As a supervisor and a therapist at the Veterans Administration Medical Center in New York City between 1975 and 1985, I supervised or treated over 40 Vietnam combat veterans suffering from PTSD and addicted to drugs and/or alcohol. After my resignation in 1985, I continued treating privately a group of patients with whom I had been working intensively during the previous several years.

These patients, in addition to the above cluster of symptoms, presented an extremely low level of social adjustment, very poor or nonexistent work history following the Vietnam War experience, and a deteriorated or nonexistent love and sex life. Some lived in a state of total isolation except for leaving their furnished room or apartment for their appointments. For some, these appointments became the only anchor to life and reality. For others, it often became impossible to maintain the link, and they would miss a number of appointments at a time.

I saw these patients in therapy from one to five times per week, often with the adjunct of group therapy. The revenge motif was continuous for these men, and was strikingly juxtaposed to their inability to mourn. In treatment, the focus on the vicissitudes of grief and mourning turned out to be of special value and yielded the most important changes in the quality of therapy and in the emotional life of these men.

This paper will deal with some specific changes I have observed during psychoanalytic psychotherapy of substance-abusing combat veterans with PTSD. These changes have to do with the gradual shift from nightmare, with its direct reference to disturbing war events, to more distorted symbolic dreams, with or without reference to the Vietnam experience. The changes in the dream content will be considered specifically in the context of working through these men's complex feelings about loss.

Usually, the motif that dominated these veterans' minds and souls when one of their buddies died was that of revenge. They did all they could to blunt the mourning process and not cry. Even for those who cried, the tears did not and could not become part of the process of mourning, but rather fueled sentiments of hatred and thoughts of revenge.

Since during combat there was much interest in maintaining a high level of war spirit, the problematic impact of what the veterans experienced often went undetected. It was not unusual for emotional breakdown to go unnoticed, especially if the content of the soldier's behavior could be interpreted as the revengeful attitude of a crazed but good soldier.

Jones (1946) pointed out that when psychiatric patients cannot be treated during the initial stages of breakdown, the prognosis becomes serious. In most cases, the seriousness of the traumatic experiences for the Vietnam combat veteran did not become manifest until long after discharge, when they appeared in the PTSD syndrome, which includes recurring nightmares.

These nightmares tend to leave the veterans very frightened for themselves and for the lives of those around them. During the nightmare experience, the veteran would often find himself in reality attacking the unaware mate sleeping next to him. The fear that these nights brought to the veteran and to his mate added an incredible strain to an already difficult relationship and to a psychic organization already in a state of great despair.

Thus, the frightening relevance of the nightmare in the lives of these men has to do not only with what the content of the nightmare keeps on reminding the dreamer of, but also with the fact that the dream, now in the present, with its overwhelming content, keeps on burdening the psychic apparatus of the dreamer, offering him no relief during his sleep and thus inflicting additional trauma to an already traumatized psyche (Eissler, 1966).

When one considers that these nightmare experiences had often gone on for many years before these men could begin talking about them, one can start appreciating the psychological state they were in when they finally entered treatment.

Adolescence, Stress, Substance Abuse, and the War

Many of the soldiers were as young as 17 when they fought in Vietnam. Blos (1968) has stressed the fact that "character formation and adolescence are synonymous." He points out that character, as the definite component of adult psychic structure, performs an essential function in mature psychic organism. This function is manifested in the maintenance of psychosomatic homeostasis, in patterned self-esteem regulation, and in the stabilization of ego identity.

In the combat veterans I have treated, psychosomatic homeostasis is nonexistent, and self-esteem lacks any reliable sense of regulation, moving from points of isolated feelings of grandiosity to the pits of uselessness, paranoia, and consequent suicidal and homicidal potential. As to the stabilization of ego identity, one is struck by these patients' relentless feeling of nonexistence, of not belonging.

This, of course, greatly influences the establishment of a therapeutic alliance and the course of therapy itself. As Musatti (1976) has pointed out, what determines the outcome of therapy is the influence of the trauma, the strength of the impulses, and the alteration of the ego. These patients had great troubles on every count.

As to the ego weakness, developmental vicissitudes are crucial. Adolescent regression in particular, with its quality of being unavoidable and obligatory (Blos, 1968), breaks down the equilibrium to the ego's disadvantage. If to this phase of specific regression one adds the fact that these young men had to deal with their adolescent feelings of change and loss along with their sexual and aggressive impulses in the context of the traumatic experience of the Vietnam war, it becomes no wonder that their ego stability and superego functions suffered greatly.

Many of these men were still living through a most important phase of identity formation. They were facing the modifications and integrations of their self and object representations. The sense of morality and the way of pursuing goals, settling disputes, and dealing with losses receive a fundamental impetus during adolescence. Yet it was during this period of development that some of these men got a very disturbing lesson in the way disputes are settled and in the way right is distinguished from wrong.

In addition, during adolescence there is a cracking of old idols, beliefs, and illusions about oneself and others. One often feels compelled to deal not only with these losses but also with the desire to deny the loss and recapture somewhat what is really inevitably lost. What many hoped the war could give them was a purpose, and also the illusion of escaping limitations.

Paradoxically, while the soldiers saw great limitations and witnessed the killing and maiming of human lives, yet with each experience and each loss they often affirmed an eventually disturbing sense of potency. They in fact knew that they would be able to take the law into their own hands and could avail themselves of a quick retribution, which was acceptable and encouraged, and which contributed to ignoring loss and human limitations.

All of these highly stressful situations landed heavily on individuals already stressed, often much more than they were willing to recognize. How were these men handling this stress? How were they affected by the stress of war that occurred at a developmentally stressful period?

It has been pointed out (Petersen & Spiga, 1982) that four elements are of crucial importance in evaluating how one handles stress: timing, preparation, vulnerability, and social support.

1) *Timing of developmental stress.* The Vietnam war, with its many traumatizing experiences, included sudden, inescapable, and almost furious combat situations. The stress of the war has not only been reported by every veteran I have worked with, but has also been amply documented in the literature (Blank, 1982; Figley, 1978; Kelly, 1985; Schwartz, 1984).

2) *Preparation.* The more one is prepared for a specific experience, the better one can cope and adapt. Yet, no matter how good their training prior to going to Vietnam, these men could never be sufficiently prepared to suddenly be shot at, to see friends crippled and killed, to witness or be part of atrocities to soldiers or civilians. They could never be sufficiently prepared to walk in the jungle not knowing who the enemy was, when he would suddenly appear, or when he would manifest his presence via traps and ambushes.

3) *Individual level of vulnerability.* This is an important factor in general and was particularly important in Vietnam. It is related to existing developmental deficits that are inevitably reactivated in situations of stress, and it also has to do with current conscious and unconscious processes. Greenacre (1967), for instance, has said that whenever a traumatic experience is associated with an underlying fantasy, the fixation on the trauma is usually quite severe.

Thus, if there had been castration fears, the contact with bodies of mutilated and dead soldiers could reactivate that fear, making the trauma even more entrenched (Rosenberg, 1945). While this fear could somewhat be defended against by reaction formation and identification with the aggressor during the war, because of the level of existing ego weakness and the severity of the ongoing trauma, the ego became more prone to become overwhelmed and unable to provide for itself adequate defensive organization.

Jacobson (1964) has pointed out that the sense of self-esteem becomes greatly affected when there is disharmony between the self representation and the wishful concept of the self. Many of these combat veterans wished to see themselves as capable, sought after, in control, and with unlimited ability and freedom to act and react. To some extent, this had been the way they had seen themselves in Vietnam. When they came home, many had to balance that wishful sense of self against their actual experience of themselves as incapable, unwanted, and limited in their ability to influence a reality they often saw as either uncaring or openly hostile.

As Rochlin (1973) has suggested, everything that lowers self-esteem increases aggression. This has been so for those veterans who had been exposed to the trauma of combat and whose present emotional state touched off existing still-undifferentiated levels of ego organization. In these cases, the impact of earlier developmental traumas and conflicts and of the later war traumas overwhelmed the ego in such a way that it became extremely difficult to utilize defenses or influence drives (Reich, 1960). The clinical and human picture was one of men who felt very vulnerable, who oscillated between withdrawal from the world and desire for a hostile destructive and retaliatory contact, and who felt at times like puppets whose strings were being pulled by everyone except themselves.

4) The last of the four elements regarding the impact of stress has to do with the presence and value of *social support*. Often many of the combat veterans found it impossible to utilize the outside world for the purpose of eventually transforming traumas into components of their evolving character formation. Not only had their cumulative traumatic experiences been overwhelming, but the outside world was distancer and judge, rather than friendly welcomer. The veteran was left alone to deal with all that was frightening and unbearable. He continuously oscillated between withdrawal and rageful feelings and reactions, thus avoiding the internal confrontation with himself and, with it, any potential for resolution.

The way a person will be able to cope with what comes his way is determined not only by the quality of internalized values, beliefs, and objects, but also by the maturity of the internalized representations and structure, along with other psychosexual, cognitive, and interpersonal developments (Spero, 1986). For the combat veterans I treated, the sense of values, and the belief and trust in themselves and others during earlier times of development, were often confusing and unreliable. They generally needed to split the good from the bad, thus preserving a semblance of object relationships that sacrificed sense of self and honesty for the need to be loved (Menaker, 1979), real self to the development of false self (Winnicott, 1965). This splitting fostered the development of a personality that felt basically victimized but that was inevitably prone to rage reactions experienced as frightening emotional breakdowns triggered by self-object failure (Kohut, 1972).

These reactions, in a personality that had grown up with the kind of self and object representations described above, now found a peculiar expression in the context of the war zone. Here the frustrated, unempathically responded to, grandiose child was given an opportunity, not to mature and change, but to grow up in its original pathological way. It is like witnessing a psychotic person who goes into a manic-like episode or period. He wants to convince himself and others it is the expression of strength, while it really is the expression of needs, impulses, and desires that come out of an extremely impoverished ego and that, in the absence of a mature superego, overwhelm the ego, leaving it unable to organize defenses and finally crushing it under their own strength.

In the context of overwhelming impulses and experiences, the use of drugs and alcohol often served a purpose that, to some extent, was similar to the revenge behavior while in Vietnam. It gave the veteran the appearance of organizing and giving meaning to a life that otherwise seemed meaningless and dominated and controlled by everybody else. In Vietnam the sense of powerlessness and of being at the mercy of situations that one could not control or understand received a semblance of meaning by reducing the complexity into the single, structured intent of seeking revenge. Back home the use of drugs and alcohol became that apparently simple and structured behavior, around which life became organized, and which was used to recapture a semblance of control. It became a compelling behavior that greatly contributed to denying fears and limitations and to avoiding dealing with the more difficult tasks of mourning and growing up.

It seems to me important in this context to note that the timing of drug use was far from uniform among these patients. Some men had never used drugs until their tour of duty in Vietnam. Others had used drugs before they went to Vietnam, but almost totally abstained while in Vietnam, and then resumed drug use while in the war, waiting to be sent home. Still others never used drugs before or during the military service, but began using drugs shortly after returning home, when they felt trapped by the stereotyped responses of their civilian countrymen curious about the number of killings and the like. They found themselves unable to integrate the recent war experience in the context of their rediscovered shaky sense of self.

Though differing in the timing of their drug use, these patients have in common a pervasive feeling of loneliness, emptiness, and depression, along with intense feelings of rage and vengefulness touched off by narcissistic hurt. Wurmser (1981) postulates that in order to defend themselves from the impact of these feelings whenever limitations are imposed, drugs are used in order to eliminate or reduce feelings of: 1) rage for the impaired limitations; 2) shame for having had their impotent, threatened, and weak self exposed; and 3) hurt and rejection at the realization that the "other person" is not as great, redeeming, or giving as hoped for.

In the patients we are considering, the "other person" became identified not only with members of their families and with girlfriends, but also with the government of the United States and the whole country. Even for those who did not start using drugs until after Vietnam, and who had felt valued and accepted for their performance in combat, drug use contains a transferential response to their country. For them, the USA had become the parent who first seduced them into feeling accepted, who invited them in the sharing of its power, but who then left them alone to confront their limitations, their loneliness, and their rage at the perceived abandonment.

In this context, the drug use is not only "a replacement for a defect in the psychological structure" (Kohut, 1971, p. 46) of these men; it also indicates a deficit in the quality of their internalized object relationships, which get reactivated in connection with persistent traumatic situations and which speak to the intensity of their aggressive feelings, to the weakness of their ego, and to defects of superego structure.

Drugs then become a "surrogate ideal, a substitute value—which would normally be supplied by the internal sense of meaning, goal directedness and value orientation" (Wurmser, 1981, p. 148). In addition, given the vulnerability of these patients to the impact of their rage reactions, the drugs also provide an opportunity for a semblance of control, which includes an illusory reassurance about their feelings of castration, while at the same time they actually remain the impotent and castrated children they felt they had to be.

While in Vietnam, the rage reactions that had a developmental antecedent received a powerful additional impetus from the enemy of the country, which in turn became a personal enemy toward whom rage could be directed and expressed. On the other hand, these men also felt much rage toward the government as the ideal that failed to sustain them in the aftermath of the Vietnam experience.

As this paper will continue to show, rage and vengefulness were predominant feelings in these combat veterans. Thus it became imperative that these feelings could be valued and understood in the treatment situation so that they could slowly give way to the process of mourning.

On Nightmares

Hartmann (1984) has pointed out that nightmares are long, vivid, frightening dreams which awaken the sleeper and whose content is usually clearly recollected. Post-traumatic nightmares are described by the same author as dreams in which the dreamer is led straight back to traumatic events or experiences with no or very few associations. Rado (1942) considered nightmares a prominent symptom of traumatic war neurosis.

Some authors have associated nightmares with a high level of anxiety (Hersen, 1972), with overly dependent relationships with parents (Fairbairn, 1952), and with a great fear about death (Fedelman & Hersen, 1967). Freud (1920) thought that nightmares represent fulfillment of superego wishes and that they are a response to guilt feelings and a wish for punishment. Jones (1931) thought that nightmares represent a compromise formation between sexual and incestuous wishes.

In considering the post-Vietnam syndrome, Sudak and colleagues (1984) have concluded that wartime experiences activate premorbid conflicts. Post-traumatic psychopathology is viewed as a failure to cope with revived conflicts. Lidzt (1946) found that nightmares appeared subsequent to a soldier's loss of emotionally significant persons.

Nightmare is thus a symptom of the trauma and a communication about the trauma. Kanzer (1955) says that though the dream is a narcissistic and intrapsychic phenomenon, there are communicative elements in it, and that to communicate the dream to another person is in itself a continuation of the tendency within the dreamer to establish contact with the reality.

We see here two important and crucially interrelated phenomena: the nightmare and the communication of its content to another person, specifically the therapist. In all the combat veterans I have worked with, for a long time since their inception, the nightmares existed without being shared with anybody else. The traumatized veteran, who often had lost a sense of basic trust in himself and the world, experienced the nightmares as additional attacks by ghosts he could not put to rest. As mentioned earlier, the dream itself began to have a traumatic effect on the dreamer, who would at times find himself waking up in the process of attacking the mate who was next to him.

Yet recalling combat experiences in nightmares also served the purpose of maintaining a connection to people and situations that could not be let go of. Fox (1974) spoke of aggression in soldiers following the death of a buddy in combat. He found a relationship between psychiatric difficulties subsequent to combat (including nightmares) and narcissistic injury and rage. In therapy he found that "the predominant theme was one of revenge rather than mourning" (p. 808). He concluded that the loss of buddies represented a narcissistic injury with resultant threat to the self accompanied by rage and retaliatory actions.

Can the nightmare itself also contain an attempt to traumatically master a traumatic situation? Can the nightmare represent an attempt to keep on giving some sense, thought painful and distorted, to a self that feels purposeless and continuously prone to feelings of fragmentation and nonexistence? I respond affirmatively to both questions. Once the veteran began to find a way of sharing in therapy the frightening content of his nightmares and the memories of combat stimulated by the nightmares, he found, in the emotionally overwhelming recollection of those events, a new chance of mastering the trauma and dealing with losses.

It seems to me that the combat veteran with and in the nightmare tried to deal with at least three things: 1) to own a part of his life that he could not dissociate himself from without creating an unfillable gap in his emotional and historical development and continuity of his sense of self; 2) to deal with the rage that he felt toward the family for having left him so exposed and unprotected during and after the war; and 3) to set in motion a process of mourning that could include ambivalence even toward those buddies who had been killed in action. The combat veteran in fact had been aware only of feelings of attachment toward those soldiers who had died, and of feelings of hatred and revenge toward the enemy. During the process of mourning, he could begin to experience guilt for wishing to survive, and he could begin to mourn not only the dead comrades but also other previously unmourned losses.

Let us now discuss the treatment of two combat veterans in order to illustrate the theoretical points discussed above and to point out some specific treatment issues as they relate to nightmares and mourning.

The Case of Mr. G

I started seeing Mr. G in individual sessions shortly after he entered the drug program where I was working. He was 34 years old at that time and was living a totally withdrawn life. Except for a man 25 years his senior, he had no contacts with anyone outside the clinic. His parents were both dead. He had one sister he had not talked to since his discharge from the service. His older friend visited him a few times a week for a couple of hours at a time and did food shopping for him. The only time Mr. G left his apartment was to go to the clinic and to go to church on Sunday.

He reported having upsetting nightmares every night. These nightmares, besides being replicas of actual experiences in Vietnam, were also often scenes of comrades' dead bodies calling his name. Mr. G felt that he too should be dead. At times he felt as if he were dead, and that the dead comrades were telling him that he belonged with them.

Mr. G was the only son in a family of Western European background. He had one sister two years younger whom he had not seen or spoken to in about ten years. His mother died when he was eight years old, and his father died while he was completing his tour of duty in Vietnam.

When Mr. G was 14 years old, his father married a woman the patient disliked, and who, he felt, manipulated the father into leaving his estate to her to the exclusion of his children. After his mother's death, Mr. G lived with an aunt, and he never felt welcome at his father's house. Yet he maintained an idealized image of his father as a hard-working man and a loving father who just happened to fall in the hands of a seductive and manipulative woman.

During adolescence, Mr. G got often into fist fights, and on a couple of occasions he spent the night in jail. His feelings toward significant others in his life were characterized by guilt for his mother's death (if he had been a good boy she would have lived longer), rage and a wish for revenge toward his stepmother, a tendency to protect his father and distance himself from any feelings of anger toward him, and ambivalence toward his sister and brother-in-law who had given up on him during the time when, after discharge from the army, he had gotten heavily into drugs.

He had not used any drugs in Vietnam, but he began using heroin a few months after discharge. Then he also started abusing pills and alcohol.

In treatment he developed a strong attachment to the therapist. He felt understood for the first time, though he remained cautious about revealing details of his Vietnam experience. As the sense of trust increased, he began recounting some of the horrors, including killing, mutilating, and tasting the enemy's blood. At the same time, he reported that nightmares were increasing in frequency and intensity. He was sleeping less and becoming afraid to fall asleep.

Later on in group, he was not sure that he could be specific about some of his experiences in Vietnam. He feared that he would be judged as crazy and thus rejected by his own friends (who in reality had been involved in very similar experiences). The focus in treatment was to provide an atmosphere where he would feel safe and dependent, and where his feelings about losses from Vietnam and reaching all the way back to his childhood could begin to be dignified.

As this possibility started to become a reality, a number of shifts took place in the life of Mr. G. His drug use decreased and then stopped altogether (he has not used drugs for the last four years). He began doing his shopping by himself. He started going out of his furnished room more often. In addition, his dream content began to change. During the last couple of years he began to daydream about a job and about a girl. He had not been with a girl since shortly after discharge from Vietnam.

As for the shift in the dream content, he reported, for instance, that he had again dreamed of the dead soldiers calling his name. Yet this time it was not frightening. The voices seemed less eerie, almost soothing while calling out his name.

In discussing the patient's longing for the dead person, Volkan (1981) has said that the patient also wishes to kill in order to complete the work of mourning. What seems relevant in this context is the attempt at mastery implicit in these forms of communication with the dead. Here, besides the content of the dream and its attached affect, what seemed relevant was that this dream had taken place during my vacation. As we talked about it, Mr. G became sad and spoke of how much he had missed me. He said that often when he was alone he would call my name, which he found soothing.

So one element of the dream was the need for reversal. He was the one calling me wishing to be with me. He was the psychologically dead person calling out in order to be allowed to come back and live. The other part of the reversal was the affect. He was not only sad and desperate, he was also angry at me for having left him.

Now for the first time he could accept my interpretation and acknowledge that he had been angry with me. Yet how difficult it was for him to show anger to the people he loves and needs. He would have liked to yell at me to come back, but he was afraid that I would be put off by that, so he had to show only the grateful part.

As we continued dealing with all of these feelings, he reported the following brief dream. "I dreamt that I was helping prevent somebody from getting killed with a lethal injection." His associations related to injections used to make people tell the truth. Here, besides some implicit homosexual concerns, which were not touched on at this time, we dealt with what he feared might be secrets extracted from him against his will. It was, in a sense, his way of saying that he was readier than he had been in a long time to approach the subject of secrets.

Secrets here related mostly to his relationship with his sister and the incestuous wishes he had been harboring toward her. He was able to express longing for her, but also, slowly, ambivalence and rage at her for what he perceived as her abandoning him after his discharge from Vietnam when he got heavily into drugs and alcohol.

The impact on his emotional life of his feelings of rage could now be discussed in terms of his relationship with his sister, his childhood history, and his Vietnam experience, where he had dealt with his rage by killing and destroying. We also paid attention to his confusing present emotional state, where rage felt overwhelming and with no chance of acceptable resolution.

This of course has been and still is far from simple. For instance, as Mr. G began to feel comfortable looking more in depth at his relationship with his father, he had to face the painful realization that his youth, his longings, and his needs had been killed off during his teens by his father's emotional blindness and unavailability. To mourn not only his father's death, but also his absence and rejection while he was still alive, has been a profoundly difficult experience in treatment. Yet it has also allowed him to start mourning his own sense of unrealistic omnipotence and to begin to move toward less frantic, action-oriented behavior.

Two recent dreams testify to his increased commitment to more emotional truth. The first was: "I was fighting with my father. I was kicking the shit out of him." The second dream was: "There was an army officer. He was telling me that I had not been treating children well. I denied it. Then a friend came over. I asked if you had sent him to me. He said yes. I felt hopeful for a moment, but then the officer took me away anyway."

In his associations, memories of wishing his father dead when he was a young teenager were recalled with much affect. He remembered how scared he was of his thoughts, and that he would then go at night to his father's bed and listen to his breathing to make sure that he was still alive. As for the second dream, he thought that maybe he was the child wanting to tell his father that he (the father) had not treated him well. Yet he is scared of asserting his feelings. He fears that he either will kill the father, as he is doing in the first dream, or will be taken out of circulation, as is happening in the second dream. So he wants my protection. Except that he is not sure that I will really be there. He is also not sure that without my actual presence he can make it.

The fear of the loss of the therapist is a continuous concern among these combat veteran patients once they have established a strong emotional bond. They do not believe that anyone will really stick around long enough. They seem at times convinced that their needs, their craziness, their demands, and their history will drive anybody away. So they keep on testing, keep on doubting, keep on provoking abandonment.

Yet by doing so, they also try to do over again, and possibly better this time, the developmental stage of separation and rapprochement. The hope on their part is that when they come back to the therapist with their "bad parts," the therapist will accept them back, thus supporting the expression of their individual and separate feelings, and will communicate that the rapprochement and the refueling will still be possible.

The Case of Mr. B

Mr. B came into treatment following an explosive episode at home in which he threatened first to blow up his parents' home and then to kill himself. He was hospitalized on a psychiatric ward for five weeks and then discharged back to the drug clinic, where he had already been a patient for several months because of his drug addiction. He was very guarded, suspicious of my motives, and sure that I would not understand "a damn thing about Vietnam."

The first few months of treatment were a testing period, with the focus on his feelings toward me and therapy, along with his perception of and reaction to his current family situation. He had been divorced for some time. He was living at his parents' house, and he was unemployed.

The discussion about his life in the present led us to talking in great detail about his cocaine use. As we tried to understand the effect cocaine had on him, he revealed that usually during the cocaine high he talked a lot about Vietnam. It was as if cocaine had become the facilitator, the enabler for his need to verbalize combat experiences without the inhibitions present in his sober state.

At the same time, he began reporting nightmares which, he said, he had been having for several years. These nightmares were filled with scenes of dismembered bodies, shelling, ambushes, shooting, and screaming. He slowly began talking about Vietnam. A few months later he also joined the therapy group of combat veterans that I was leading.

As with other combat veterans during the next several months, the transference slowly evolved from guarded and suspicious to positive. Yet there was a noticeable split. I was good and the rest of the world was bad. He felt that he could count on me, and to some extent on the other group members, who were then related to in the same way each had related to other selected GIs during Vietnam, with closeness and sense of mutual protection.

Though Mr. B had been erratic in his attendance at the group meetings during the first several months, he now became committed and reliable. He became the one who usually initiated confrontation when another group member missed a session.

These confrontations provided an opportunity in vivo to see also how some of these men dealt with frustration, doubt, and rage. On a few occasions the level of verbalized rage became so intense that the existing loyalty to each other turned temporarily into a paranoid perception of the other, which seemed to destroy anything positive that had existed before.

As distressing as these sessions could become, they also became for Mr. B and other patients opportunities to confront and try to understand the impact that similar situations in the past had had on them. Also, inasmuch as sessions of this emotional intensity could be put in a context that did not allow easy self-righteousness, they opened up the possibility to see life not as a sum of paranoid and dangerous expectations, but as an inevitable series of falls and recuperations.

As for Mr. B, he spoke vividly of how the rage at the enemy was dealt within Vietnam. In a poignant, and at times apparently disorganized manner, he would go back and forth between Vietnam and the present, expressing in the process rage at the "system" that he now felt was trying to tie his hands, while in Vietnam that same "system" had given him license to do anything he wanted with those same hands.

When, after about two years of working with him, I decided to leave the clinic, feelings of abandonment, longing, and rage began to make their appearance, first weakly and then more with directness and strength. They were only mildly mitigated by my reassuring him that I would continue working with him and the rest of the group privately.

During the first month of seeing me in my private office, he reported his first dream not related to Vietnam. The dream was: "I came for a group session and the group members told me that they had a surprise for me. They took me to your old room at the clinic, and there you were. You had come back to the clinic."

The new situation, with its limitations of more strictly assigned time and his and other patients' inability to just drop in, gave a further impetus to the need to deal more in depth with issues of loss. The dream made it more comfortable for Mr. B to begin to express his attachment to me, the tension he felt about it, and the ways he would try to deny or dilute both his longings and his feelings of deprivation. He could also begin to see that, hidden in his expressions of rage, there was much hurt and pain.

The motif of loss and mourning continued to occupy many individual and group sessions. It extended to Vietnam of course, but also slowly began to include, for Mr. B, the profound, painful, and unfulfilled longing for his mother. At the same time, it brought to the surface his hate for women he sought for their ability to soothe him and make him feel safe, but whom he hated because they made him feel weak, vulnerable, and dependent, and thus exposed to renewed fear of abandonment.

Mr. B continued reporting dreams that, though still containing elements related to the Vietnam experience, also seemed to open the door to richer understanding of his life prior to Vietnam. A few months after the dream about my office, he told the following dream: "I had a submachine gun. There were many people in black pajamas. I let them go as they jumped through a window. Then a naked woman came into the room. She too was about to go, but I wanted her to stay. She jumps off the window but I grab her by her tits. Her tits stretched as she reached the ground. I could hold her no longer. I got mad and opened fire. I woke up in a sweat."

He associated people with black pajamas with the Viet Cong. He wished that he could finally forget about them and Vietnam. Yet now, as when he was in Vietnam, he needed help. He remembered how often, while he was in Vietnam, he had hoped to have a strong woman by his side who would protect him. His thoughts went to his mother. Desires of an oedipal nature became complicated by feelings of sadness and anger at her. He recalled an unlovable, punitive, distant, and "milkless" mother, who had also been capable of moments of tenderness and affection during his childhood. The alternating of these two conflicting levels of relatedness and created much ambivalence in Mr. B. He felt seduced into a profound desire to abandon himself in his mother's lap only to then feel lonely, abandoned, and frustrated at the precarious hold that he had on his mother's presence.

This period in treatment was one of confusion, yet growth. He tried to own up to the pain and ambivalence of his early relationship with his mother without immediately needing to reassure himself by enumerating the good things that she had been able to do for him during the last several years. He began to appreciate his demands and his needs without feeling compelled to act in such a way as to compromise the dignity of those needs and thus in the end make them look as bad as the acting out behavior was.

Inasmuch as he was now able to stay with the pain, he did not have to camouflage it with impulsive expressions of rage or with destructive and self-destructive behavior. Of course, by eliminating much of the acting out, his depression became more visible, and he experienced his dependence on me as more necessary, but also more anxiety provoking due to homosexual fears and expectations of humiliation and loss.

As necessary as it was to look at these feelings, they also provoked temporary periods of paranoia and rage. For instance for a while he found it extremely difficult to ride the subway because he felt that people were looking at him and making fun of him. In these instances, he would place himself strategically with his back against the subway car door as if ready to counter the enemy's attack.

The investigation of these situations led to a better understanding of his current life events and of related experiences in Vietnam. We discovered that the period of subway phobia was taking place in the context of difficulties that he was having with his girlfriend, who had thrown him out of her apartment following a night when he almost strangled her while he was having a nightmare related to Vietnam. As we probed further, we learned that the nightmare and its related incident with his girlfriend had taken place around the same time of the year when, many years before in Vietnam, he had in fact strangled a Vietnamese girl who was about to shoot one of his friends.

Reliving experiences such as this often adds to the existing potential for regression and defensive posture. Yet, in general, Mr. B seems to have gotten stronger in his newfound courage to look more honestly at his relationship with his family, his insecurity, his vulnerability, his developmental losses, and the losses he suffered in Vietnam. He has begun to show a more consistent wish to live. On an existential level, he has been able to take responsibility for the pursuit of some goals that he would previously have abandoned quickly in the face of even minor hurdles and then felt angry at the system for not giving him a chance.

He also has not used cocaine or other drugs for more than a year, and he is more committed to talking than to acting out. Though this is, in itself, a remarkable achievement, it also leaves a person like Mr. B, who has been so dependent on the organizing potential of the drugs, vulnerable to the new commitment to tolerate and grow within a more realistic sense of himself and others.

Further Treatment Considerations

I would like to say a few words about my input in the treatment in order to expand on what was already presented in the case histories.

Especially during the first few months of treatment, I facilitated the sense of safety for these men by being at times more verbally active than I usually am. This was done for the purpose of inviting connectedness, not to block away recollection of painful material. In fact, I backed off quickly once the patients began talking, and I was ready to pick up on their reaction to my being quiet in order to explore feelings of paranoia, mistrust, and abandonment.

Neutrality has usually not been on my priority list with these patients, and my verbal communication has at times included the use of curse words along the line of their own usage. My verbal activity has been a way of acknowledging that their silence and their reluctance were actually filled with an intensity that often frightened them, but that nonetheless they needed to familiarize themselves with.

One, of course, has to be alert to countertransference manifestations. In order not to hear very disturbing material, the therapist can push these patients out of treatment. The therapist can then explain the outcome of treatment on the basis of the patient's resistance as supposedly manifested by his inability to be introspective, his missing appointments, or his coming late to sessions. The same goal of the therapist not to hear overwhelming war material can be reached by talking too much, be being too directive, and by thus not allowing the veteran to feel safe enough to share difficult experiences and feelings.

Countertransference is also present when the therapist begins to feel that he can be the powerful omnipotent parent who will solve the patient's problems and save him from the horrible world that he is in. Given the potential presence of the therapist's own unresolved feelings about rage and mourning, along with the presence of complex political feelings regarding a war that affected every segment of the population, it is no wonder that countertransference can be a hindrance to treatment process and outcome or, with acknowledgment, a powerful tool to pave the way for the resolution of difficult feelings in the patient and in the therapist himself.

It is as if the war continues in the treatment situation, and the therapist is asked to join in fighting the multifaceted enemy that lives in the intrapsychic life of these men and in his own. And so, while this intensity is dignified and pursued, one must remain alert to the need for separateness, so that verbal action in treatment can be used to facilitate, not choke the process of mourning.

These patients came to treatment feeling chained to a terrifying, yet for them valuable and important past. They came to treatment feeling prisoners of a war that had touched them and gotten deep inside their bodies and souls. They had reached a point where hallucinatory processes were often present, with disturbing breaks with reality and sudden though temporary total immersion in the past (Vietnam). I had to allow them to take me along on their journey, while at the same time communicating that I wanted them to live, that this was an important and difficult fight that they could not do on their own, and that it was OK to rely on each other and on me.

This was expanded in the sense of valuing their need for protection and assistance, while appreciating the lack of protection they had suffered in the past, the sense of vulnerability they often felt exposed to, and the not unusual tendency to behave in a counterphobic way in order to deny their fears and their vulnerability. What was also stressed was that the goal of treatment was not for me to take away the pain or cancel the past, but for them to learn what had made it impossible for them to dignify the value of human presence as an aid in the experience of pain. We thus tried to learn what in the present prevented them from looking at me and people close to them in such a fashion.

Clearly developmental considerations were kept in mind throughout. Yet neutrality, as mentioned earlier, was not of primary concern. Given the depth of their suspiciousness, the unusual nature of their combat experiences, and their level of rage, their sense of victimization and depression, a neutral person is at best a useless person who does not even facilitate some approximation of human connectedness in the presence of emotionally devastating communication. Some of these veterans looked at Vietnam as a huge mortuary, and they now went through their civilian life as if always in the presence of death.

Finally there is the issue of substance abuse. Elsewhere (Smaldino, 1983) I have stressed the value of looking at substance abuse as a vehicle for a better understanding of the patients' language and life story. Having to deal with patients with a history of action-oriented behavior, and a present tendency for action through continued drugs and alcohol use, can be overwhelming for the therapist. Feeling responsible for the lives of these patients, the therapist may feel compelled to request that they stop using drugs, and to make this the sine qua non for the continuation of treatment. The fact is that this rigid stance is usually useless and unproductive, and sets the stage for a premature closure to any meaningful communication and/or treatment.

It seems to me that these patients are basically asking the therapist to be willing to get his hands dirty, to be willing to fight with them and stay in the fight. The request, followed by frustration and threats, that the patient stop using drugs is usually seen by the patient as the therapist's rule that the patient stop all the "crazy behavior" and get down to the business of change. The result inevitably is a conviction on the part of the patient that if the therapist does not want his "crazy behavior" and cannot cope with it, he also does not want and cannot cope with the patient himself.

Often a nonjudgmental and curious concern about the value and experience of drug use can, in time, bring about the kind of discovery that can yield important results, even in the area of substance abuse. This is not to say that one has to avoid discussing reality issues connected to the abuse of drugs and alcohol. It means that one has to be open to seeing this aspect of these patients' lives as a compellingly difficult behavior that also contains adaptive elements worth discovering, so that through this, too, the process of mourning and authenticity can proceed and be more fully appreciated.

Final Remarks

In discussing the progression from nightmare to dream, from hopelessness to possibility, in Vietnam veterans, some points should be stressed in conclusion. The depth of the material regarding the combat experiences must be faced in the context of the entire person, present and past. As much as the therapist should not insist that this particular material be pursued relentlessly, he must be willing to enter a territory which, no matter what the diagnosis, is compelling and influential.

The therapist must be willing to approach, withstand, and at times introduce a level of intensity that can pave the way for the patient to begin to belong to himself and to the present. The knowledge that one can never go back and redo events and traumas can be unbearable to face. It is a testimony to the strength of some of these patients, as it is to the strength of many who suffered excruciating traumas, that they are willing and able to move beyond the tragic loss of part of their lives.

Finally, it has to be a humbling experience to work with these patients, since one is sometimes placed in the role of witness to something that at times seems too terrible to be put into words. When words can finally be connected to feelings of traumatic experiences in the context of an intense treatment relationship, there comes the further task of mourning. The veteran no longer personified by the magic and heroism of action and feels bereft of the past sense of importance.

Despite all the obstacles and limitations described, many patients yearn for the permission to feel like a human being among human beings. Ultimately, as in all treatment relationships, how therapy proceeds will be affected by the fears and conflicts that the intimacy of the therapeutic human connection evokes.

References

Blank, A. S., Jr. (1982). Stresses of war: The example of Vietnam. In L. Goldberger & S. Breznitz (Ed.), *Handbook of stress: Theoretical and clinical aspects* (pp. 631–643). New York: Free Press.

Blos, P. (1968). Character formation in adolescence. *Psychoanalytic Study of the Child, 23,* 245–263.

Eissler, K. R. (1966). A note on trauma, dream anxiety and schizophrenia. *Psychoanalytic Study of the Child, 21,* 17–50.

Fairbairn, W. R. D. (1952). The war neuroses: Their nature and significance. In *Psychoanalytic studies of the personality* (pp. 256–280). London: Rutledge, Kegan & Paul.

Fedelman, M. J., & Hersen, M. (1967). Attitudes toward death in nightmare subjects. *Journal of Abnormal Psychology, 72,* 421–425.

Figley, C. R. (1978). (Ed.). *Stress disorders among Vietnam veterans: Theory, research and treatment.* New York: Brunner/Mazel.

Fox, R. (1974). Narcissistic rage and the problem of combat aggression. *Archives of General Psychiatry, 31,* 807–811.

Freud, S. (1920). Beyond the pleasure principle. *Standard Edition, 18,* 7–66.

Greenacre, P. (1967). The influence of infantile trauma in genetic patterns. In S. Furst (Ed.), *Psychic trauma* (pp. 108–153). New York: Basic Books.

Hartman, E. (1984). *The nightmare: The psychology and biology of terrifying dreams.* New York: Basic Books.

Hersen, M. (1972). The nightmare behavior: A review. *Psychological Bulletin, 78,* 37–48.

Jacobson, E. (1964). *The self and the object world.* New York: International Universities Press.

Jones, E. (1931). *On nightmares.* London: Hogarth Press.

Jones, E. (1946). Psychology and war conditions. *The yearbook of psychoanalysis* (Vol. 2, p. 174). New York: International Universities Press.

Kanzer, M. (1955). The communicative function of the dream. *International Journal of Psychoanalysis, 36,* 260–266.

Kelly, W. E. (1985). *Post-traumatic stress disorder and the war veteran patient.* New York: Brunner/Mazel.

Kohut, H. (1972). Thoughts on narcissism and narcissistic rage. *Psychoanalytic Study of the Child, 27,* 360–400.

Kohut, H. (1971). *The analysis of the self.* New York: International Universities Press.

Lidzt, R. (1946). Nightmare and the combat neuroses. *Psychiatry, 9,* 37–49.

Menaker, E. (1979). Masochism: A defense reaction of the ego. In L. Lerner (Ed.), *Masochism and the emergent ego.* New York: Human Sciences Press.

Musatti, C. (1976). *Riflessioni sul Pensiero Psicoanalitico.* Torino: Boringhieri.

Petersen, A., & Spiga, R. (1982). Adolescence and stress. In *Handbook of Stress,* L. Goldberger & S. Breznitz (Eds.), (pp. 515–520). New York: Free Press.

Rado, S. (1942). Pathodynamics and treatment of traumatic war neurosis. *Yearbook of Psychoanalysis, 1,* 203–214.

Reich, A. (1960). *Pathological forms of self-esteem regulation in psychoanalytic contributions.* New York: International Universities Press.

Rochlin, G. (1973). *Man's aggression: The defense of the self.* Boston: Gambit.

Rosenberg, E. (1945). A clinical contribution to the psychopathology of the war neurosis. *Yearbook of Psychoanalysis, 1,* 237–255.

Schwartz, H. (1984). *Psychotherapy of the combat veteran.* New York: SP Medical & Scientific Books.

Smaldino, A. (1983). From action to reflection: New depths in psychotherapy with drug addicts. *Clinical Social Work Journal, 11*(2), 151–163.

Spero, M. (1986). Aspects of identity development among Nuveau religious patients. *Psychoanalytic Study of the Child, 41,* 406.

Sudak, H., Martin, R., Corradi, R., & Gold, F. (1984). Antecedent personality factors and the post-Vietnam syndrome: Case reports. *Military Medicine, 149,* 550–554.

Winnicott, D. W. (1965). Ego distortions in terms of true and false self. In *The maturational process and the facilitating environment.* New York: International Universities Press.

Wurmser, L. (1981). Psychoanalytic considerations of the etiology of compulsive drug use. In H. Shaffer and M. E. Burglass (Eds.), *Classic contributions in the addictions,* (pp. 133–153). New York: Brunner/Mazel.

Myths, Questions, and Controversies in Work with Alcoholics

Joshua F. Cohen, M.S.

A myth attaching to therapists who work with alcoholics and alcoholism is that they are themselves alcoholics, may be the relatives of alcoholics, or somehow have suffered directly as the result of someone's alcoholism. As for me, in 1958 I had just finished a four-year training program at the Chicago Institute for Psychoanalysis in work with children and adolescents. I wanted to continue the work for which I was trained, but was looking for a chance to extend my practice to work with adults. At about this time I found a part-time job working with alcoholics under the supervision of one of the analysts trained at the Institute. So it began for me.

Of my colleagues and supervisees from then to now, so far as I know, few came from the groups encompassed by the myth.

How could this myth have gained currency? Perhaps because Alcoholics Anonymous, in which much work with alcoholics occurs, was founded by alcoholics and is an organization for alcoholics. Certainly a number of people working with alcoholics are alcoholics who no longer drink. But whatever one might speculate about the origins of the myth, the more important question is "What is its impact upon treatment?"

It is rare that a therapist working with alcoholics is not, at some time, accused of not being able to understand/know/treat/feel with or for the patient, the patient's problems, or alcoholics in general, since

51

the therapist is not personally an alcoholic. This often occurs early in the treatment. The anxious therapist accepts the myth, falls into a defensive position manifested by confession to shortcomings, or attempts to convince the patient that it isn't so, it doesn't matter, or that the accusation reflects the patient's resistance, ambivalence, or whatever. The more secure therapist, less burdened by the myth, may seek to assess this sort of attack within whatever context is appropriate, but initially can confine his or her reaction to remarks that will allow the patient (who may be threatened by the therapy, elements of the transference, or the like) the luxury of the attack in ways that might move the patient closer to a treatment alliance.

A fundamental concern at such times is not only to look at the patient and assess what he or she is saying, but to examine one's own reactions, especially countertransferential aspects, and be ready to understand what is involved and get on with whatever is to come. Should the protests continue about the therapist's deficits by virtue of not being an alcoholic, one has further opportunity to determine patterns of substance or of process and to use these in the interest of the treatment.

Frequently, the therapist is caught up in a conflict about whether the patient should better be in Alcoholics Anonymous or in more conventional treatment. Sometimes the question is seen as either/or, as if the two are mutually exclusive. Some therapists see it as a sine qua non that participation in psychotherapy and Alcoholics Anonymous should go together. Such undifferentiated responses are not diagnostically or therapeutically determined. To begin with, Alcoholics Anonymous and the people in it are hardly a monolith. A given group may be syntonic for one patient, dystonic for another. The same may be true of individual sponsors within AA. Rather than unequivocally endorsing or opposing Alcoholics Anonymous, which may often represent an abandonment of the field and renunciation of an important segment of the therapeutic arena, the therapist would want to assess closely what is happening. Certainly the AA group is not an entirely unknown entity. It can act as a control that gives added perspective to the therapist's view of the patient's work and family involvement and to how the patient handles the beginning and vicissitudes of relationships. Such a stance offers the therapist various opportunities to contribute to the patient. This is especially useful when the patient has attempted to distance him- or herself from treatment, for instance, the patient who disparages treatment, or family, or AA.

It may be helpful to view Alcoholics Anonymous from the perspective Freud (1921) provides. A group, he says, has the effect of making the members feel vulnerable and weak, or, conversely, comfortable and intensely powerful. Members of the group can be harsh or can become capable of the most idealistic and altruistic behavior. Ego functions are affected. This is accomplished through the agency of group contagion, which, in turn, rests upon group identification, the identification of members with one another. How does this come about? Freud posits that it occurs by virtue of the "love" the members feel toward the all-powerful leader of the group (whether represented by a person, ideal, or theme) and the presumably equal and unequivocal love the leader offers each member. The entire process can be likened to the surrender of self and idealization of the other that occurs in the process of being romantically in love.

In this light, how might we view Alcoholics Anonymous? There is a group bond, a group identity, derived from the shared alcoholism of the members. In the Twelve Steps, which are fundamental to participation in AA (Sheahan, 1979), there is an interesting splitting, which reinforces identification and gives strength to identity. To begin with, there is the admission of powerlessness over alcohol ("our lives have become unmanageable"), an excusing, liberating, and therefore strengthening solidarity. The steps continue that we "came to believe that a Power greater than ourselves could restore us to sanity" (which reflects submission to, and derivation of strength from a powerful, equally loving leader) reinforced by "a decision to turn our will and our lives over to the care of God as we understood him" (we can see here an explicit compact) leading to "a searching and fearless moral inventory of ourselves" (thus, the attainment of strength, initially through submission and confession of powerlessness, is turned not only into moral strength but active strength). The fifth step involves the setting up of a tripartite structure: "telling to God, oneself, and one other human being." Here we see a fusion with a mirroring other and an idealized other. Finally, in the twelfth step, "having had a spiritual awakening as a result of these steps" (becoming chosen, elected, getting group strength), "we tried to carry this message to alcoholics, and to practice these principles in all our affairs" (identification with the leader and development of structure, utilizing obsessive-compulsive defenses, which are erected in place of the previously unstructured, impulse-ridden behavior). So develops an attempt to emplace structure and codify previously impulse-ridden behavior, a partial substitution of reality principle gratifications for the prior pleasure (or pseudo-pleasure) principle orientation.

Thus, the sometime-success of Alcoholics Anonymous is not an accidental thing. Not to pay diagnostic attention to AA and to the patient's success or failure if involved with it, would be equivalent to ignoring what a patient feels and does in other critical relationships. Here the therapist works to get a sense not only of the perceived other but, especially, of what the patient brings and does in thought, feeling, and action to and with the relationship. In translating this to the AA experience, the therapist should consider the impact of AA on the grandiose patient, the depleted patient, the borderline patient, the highly aggressive patient, or the depressed patient. What are the vicissitudes of this and other relationships and how do they and treatment interdigitate?

Sometimes, for instance in setting up treatment groups, the vicissitudes, comforts, and demands of the prior relationship patterns are neglected. The protections of drinking are ripped away and exploration of possibly frightening new ground is undertaken without adequate support or preparation. Insufficient attention is given to the awkwardness behind the seeming gregariousness of the alcoholic and of the frequent difficulty in shifting to a therapeutic group relationship.

When I initiated outpatient group treatment in the Illinois Department of Mental Health in the early 1960s, I first screened records to determine whether a patient might be able to maintain attendance at group meetings, and whether the patient had other experiences that would indicate he or she would be neither too threatened by nor too threatening to a group. Then I first met with the patient individually. These meetings continued until I felt I had a decent sense of the patient and what he or she wanted and that he or she could at least talk with me and have some confidence that I would try to work in his or her interests. We examined ahead of time what might be expected from the group and what we each thought the patient might give to it. Moreover, each participant knew that I (or, in some instances, other therapists) would be available on an individual basis if needed. Concurrently, I would be meeting with people already in the group. The groups were open-ended. Everybody knew that a new member would join the group from time to time, and that now and again someone would "graduate" or drop out. No entrant came in by surprise, but, although I prepared the members for new participants coming into the group, this was done in a brief and general way, when the group mood was relatively calm. Thus, they and the new member could become involved in a relatively natural mutual exploration of each other and of their concerns.

In some respects the atmosphere regularly recapitulated that of a rather benign, alcohol-free local bar. There were "regulars," and when new people came in, concerns about security, status, self-image, anxiety, honesty, reciprocity, and the grand warp and woof of self and other would again and again be experienced, expressed, and examined. At times this would be done exclusively in the group. Sometimes a participant would return to, or end up in, individual treatment. With some patients, both modes of therapy took place concurrently (Schechter, 1959). Here too the determinants of mode reflect the interplay of therapeutic goals with respect to the patient, other patients in the group, the group-as-a-whole, and the interplay among them. These factors are influenced by the resources available to the therapist(s) in time, skill, and personnel.

Whether in a group or on an individual basis, the initiation of treatment will be a threat to the (quite possibly precarious) equilibrium of the patient. The patient may offer him- or herself to treatment with an excess of hope, more likely with seeming indifference or despair, and quite probably with the denial, disparagement, and projection thought to be characteristic of the alcoholic. To all of this the therapist should be attentive, and, somewhere early on, should present his or her credentials. Not primarily degrees, experience, or past successes. These can be offered, but may be threatening, if not disdained. Rather the therapist should present functional credentials, in other words, therapeutic receptivity, an initial ego-syntonic interpretation, careful and intelligent listening to the patient, and some ability to make sense of, organize, and master what he or she hears.

Interpretations should be ones that patients can accept, that will not frighten them and that offer them hope—if not in their ultimate redemption, then certainly in the care, competence, and understanding of the therapist. A good interpretation will evoke anything from agreement or affirmation to enlightenment and anticipation on the part of the patient. An appropriate first interpretation paves the way for those that are yet to come. The interpretive links may be of different sizes and come at irregular times, but an interpretive chain evolves.

Given the chanciness of the early phases of therapy, although legitimate interpretations can provide encouragement, care must be taken—especially in the face of bouts of drinking and the frustration of relatives—not to bury the patient in an avalanche of interpretations. A profusion of interpretations may reflect the therapist's anxiety more than the needs of the patient. There are tendencies to try to convince the reluctant patient through excessive demonstration. Concurrently, the therapist may feel that he or she may not get as good a chance again to make a given interpretation. A better notion is that no interpretation is the last interpretation. Under most conditions, many interpretations will be repeated, modified, and reworked at greater depth. Often interpretations that seem so well understood and so positively accepted in the therapy room will be forgotten, distorted, or subsequently rejected, sometimes by the very next session.

Various therapists and programs see drinking episodes as grounds for termination of treatment. Limiting treatment to the survivors of such a rule may improve statistics relating to the success rate or number of people subsequently completing treatment. However, this seems to me to load the deck against the patient and against the treatment. I see it as avoidance of responsible risk on the part of the therapist.

The alcoholic who has come to treatment has most likely interacted many times with significant others preliminary to drinking and subsequent to drinking. How this is dealt with in treatment will have transferential and countertransferential significance. To try, by fiat, to eliminate drinking and thus not to deal with what currently precipitates the drinking—and its consequences—mostly fails and, whether the fiat can be maintained or not, can skew or minimize, if not take the heart out of, the core of the treatment.

This is not to say that the therapist is indifferent to the patient's drinking. Rather, it emphasizes that the stance the therapist takes is based on assessment of what is happening with a given patient at different times in interaction with the patient's environment, the therapist, and the treatment process.

Similarly, with the question of whether or not the patient admits to being an alcoholic. The drinking may be seen as both an attempt to control and to abandon control. It is accompanied or abetted in many cases by the defense mechanism of denial. To insist on acknowledgment of alcoholism by the patient early on or prior to treatment does at least three potentially harmful things: 1) it may prevent the therapist from understanding the ways in which the patient uses denial; 2) it may narrow the arena in which the patient and therapist work out their therapeutic relationship; 3) and it may deprive the patient of a defense before it ought to be given up and a more effective way of dealing with self and world can take its place.

Patience on every side is needed especially if, as often happens, there are bouts of drinking early in the treatment. In this respect, the question of whether or not alcoholism is a physical disease, an allergy, or what (and certainly it is a physical disease in its last stages, accompanied by changes in metabolism, Wernicke's syndrome, Korsakov's disorder, cirrhosis of the liver) is really determined by the degree to which the answer(s) are considered a help to treatment. Let us consider: is alcoholism physiobiologically determined? Studies taking every side of this question abound. If alcoholism is a disease, physiologically determined, then surely it is unrealistic, except in a closed, protected setting, to expect the alcoholic to be able to stop drinking early in treatment, much as we might desire that he or she could.

On the other hand, some studies seem to indicate a much higher incidence of alcohol abuse among adolescents than among adults. What happens to account for the decrease in the number of alcoholics as time goes by? Have they all been jailed or the victims of suicide, homicide, or accident? Or is alcoholism a time-limited disease? If so, although at least one study purports to show that alcoholics have a life expectancy up to 14 years fewer than nonalcoholics, how is it that so many survive to old age? Might it be the survivors who are vulnerable to the "disease," while those who "recover" from the alcoholism reflect transient social or psychological phenomena? That would be a hopeful view. Or are there really a number of different kinds of alcoholism? One could spin this on and on. The fact is that with a given patient, unless the situation has deteriorated to its last stages, we cannot with certainty, posit the existence of a physical illness.

This ambiguity I see as an advantage. It allows for a shifting, multimodal perspective, it offers hope, and it allows us to work with the patient's view of what ails him or her. If the patient sees alcoholism as a disease, on the one hand, he or she is freed of responsibility for some of his or her behavior. This is both a relief and a disadvantage. It allows the patient to accept more readily aspects of the social role of the patient, which is well defined in our culture (Parsons, 1964), and it may initially ease acceptance of an alliance with the therapist. A relatively beneficent regression may be set up, which can be corrected (worked through) later. However, if the patient does not see alcoholism as a physical disease, this may be used to help examine the factors in the patient's psyche and relationships that make for difficulty (drinking or otherwise) and to increase the focus on challenging his or her behavior, understanding it, and taking responsibility for it.

From the foregoing, it seems evident that I see the beginning phases of treatment with alcoholics as, in many respects, similar to the initial phases of treatment with people having a wide range of psychological problems. A referral is made, a patient comes, problems are presented, there are attempts to engage, to get information about the present and the past, to make some beginning predictions—at least about treatability—and to begin communication in ways that might enhance therapeutic change. There may be some differences though. Treatment may be interrupted by drinking or other impulsive behavior leading to missed appointments. There may be strong attempts by the patient or his or her family to avoid treatment or to deny the need for it. The therapist may be confronted aggressively and disparaged for not sharing the (sometimes denied) illness or experience of the patient.

Much has been made of the difficulties of working with the alcoholic, but people with other presenting problems often pose their own sets of difficulties in treatment. Many of these difficulties are in the eye and the person of the beholder. For instance, if I may use as an example a virtual cliche, when I first began to work with alcoholics, I got many phone calls from them at home, often in the middle of the night. That virtually never happens now. This may be attributed to the fact that I see fewer alcoholics than I once did, or that alcoholics are changing. A more likely explanation is technology: For some people it is enough to hear the therapist's voice on the answering machine. That plus the uninterrupted message the patient leaves may suffice to hold the patient until a more convenient time. Other elements play a part in this, but the most important component, I think is that over the years I discovered that patients survived when I could not get back to them when they called at odd hours.

As with other patients, the mid-phase of treatment with alcoholics opens with a degree of realistic hope. Patient and therapist know each other better than before. By virtue of having negotiated the opening phases, it seems as if they can work well (or at least well enough) together, and perhaps they have begun to think that there will be fewer surprises. Yet there are disadvantages as well, and soon these begin to be manifest. There are surprises, and the patient or therapist may feel betrayed or demoralized by them. Some of the initial enthusiasm for the work, for the relationship, and for new gains may be dissipated. What may have before been novel, eliciting satisfaction or pleased surprise, might now seem routine. Visible gains or insight may seem less frequent and less profound. Family members and friends may begin to lose patience with the pace of treatment and lobby or even clamor for alterations in pace, shifting of foci, or termination. This is especially true if some of the acute alarms, the intense acting out, have become less frequent and problematic. Fatigue sets in, and there can be a tendency to miss or be late for appointments. There may be a greater likelihood of sessions seeming repetitive or missing the mark.

Yet this period, focused on the present but with excursions into or evocations of the past, serves to increase stability and to provide an arena for examination of patient-therapist interaction that will lead to the later phases of treatment. Disappointments are not seen as irrevocable or fatal, but rather as a part of the process with which therapeutic gains will ultimately be cemented. Here the therapist can foster defensive adaptations that can, in concert with the other work of therapy, help buffer the patient in relation to his or her drinking.

In the preceding section, I conveyed that I do not object to patients drinking during the course of therapy. Were I to object, what significance would it have? Transferential perhaps, but sources of transference abound. And what results would it produce, other than often prematurely ending the treatment? Rather, if a patient wants to try to engage in controlled drinking, my stance is, in most cases, to go along with it and see what happens. If the patient can handle it, which sometimes happens, well and good. If the patient cannot handle it, we have found that out together and can try to move toward a situation of no drinking based upon a shared perception of reality rather than upon conflict, ideology, or the hortatory efforts of the therapist.

Certain things have, or should have happened by the "end" of the mid-phase. Some initial problems may have diminished in frequency, intensity, and scope. Many transferential and countertransferential elements have been worked though. There is greater stability in emotions, actions, and in orientation to treatment. This reflects a somewhat altered and improved structural stability that makes for better predictability. With respect to problematic behavior, the patient has more foresight and some ability to act on it. The patient and therapist feel more secure about the patient's ability to cope with the world and to function independently.

If all this is true, why a final phase? Ideally, to attend to the disequilibrium that might be set up by the impending and actual separation inherent in terminating treatment; to pick up on the possibly new material that may be brought up under the circumstance of termination at this time; and to provide adequate balance between the closure and openness that should obtain with the termination of treatment. The concluding phase is oriented toward an integration of past and present in the service of what might occur in the future. It is the ability to deal more effectively with the future that is the measure of and the justification of the time, expense, and hard work of the treatment partnership. Here we may see commonality between psychodynamic work with alcoholics and psychodynamic work with people having other difficulties.

Yet other factors may prevent or hinder a successful termination. For instance, a family member may intervene. A parent may pull an adolescent or young adult out of treatment if the process or results are felt to be threatening to the family or to the parent's equilibrium.

Conversely, a difficulty that seems to manifest itself in the final phase is failure to terminate. This difficulty may derive from earlier phases and involves a prior failure to resolve transferential or countertransferential problems, inability to adequately assess what one is trying to accomplish, or questions of grandiosity or excessive anxiety. A problem of a different sort involves termination from fatigue, a drying up of resources. Sometimes this is extrinsic: age, illness, work load, the other commitments of life. Frequently the fatigue is intrinsic: as time passes, patient, therapist, or both, just get tired. Such fatigue may reflect the cumulative residue of errors made in treatment, of problems ignored, of questions to which insufficient attention was given. Here the most useful examples might best derive from an assessment of one's own practice.

The following case reflects some of what has been discussed:

The patient with whom I have worked longest began to see me in a group in 1962. For a period he was then seen in both the group and individually, then was seen almost exclusively individually until 1969. We have worked together sporadically for short periods since then, almost to the present, and might work together at some time in the future.

Although a successful executive and father of many children, the patient was a veteran of many binges, some of which would do harm to him or his family. He drank between binges as well, and the police were frequent callers at his home. When he was first seen, he had already been to and rejected several AA groups and a number of sponsors. Among salient elements in his history, he recalled that his father, sporadically successful in business, was an alcoholic. The patient had a good relationship with a sensitive, bright, and strong mother, who held her large family together.

When the patient was 12 the father took them driving, evidently when he had been drinking. Although the father was reputedly a good driver, he made an error in judgment, an accident ensued, the mother was injured, and the father, with the other children, waited at some remove from the car. The patient stayed at the car with his mother, who remained rational and conscious until she died. Initially, the patient's only recollection of this time was that he was stunned and sad. The family remained under one roof but lost cohesion, and the father seemed increasingly absent. During this period the patient began to be a drinker, but he finished high school despite lack of interest and episodes of undisciplined behavior.

He worked a bit after graduation, then married and, early in World War II, joined the Marine Corps. He served in the Pacific and was severely wounded. Upon release from service he embarked upon a career in communications, and he and his wife began to raise a family. His energy, articulateness, and interpersonal skills served him well until his decreasing ability to control his drinking began to hamper him severely at home and work.

Although he appeared still confident and relatively unconcerned, increasing pressure from the people around him, who were thrown into frequent turmoil by his behavior, led him first to try Alcoholics Anonymous and then, when that proved unsuccessful, to enter a treatment group with which I was working at Warren Clinic, a unit of the Division of Alcoholism of the Illinois Department of Mental Health. He was an enthusiastic participant in the group, but it seemed to have little initial impact on his drinking, and, again in response to external pressure, he agreed to inpatient hospitalization for a number of weeks at a downstate facility run by the Division. In general, he was a cooperative patient. Upon his release, he rejoined the group. Alcohol abuse diminished but did not cease. Later he stated that he felt that his needs and concerns went beyond what could be dealt with in the group. After some discussion, I began to see him individually, and he continued in the group.

Some months afterward, he was less involved in the group—which he had used well—and I began to see him exclusively in individual treatment. Our work dealt with current situations at work (where he began to become increasingly successful) and at home (where, at best, he maintained the status quo). As needed, we shuttled back and forth to and from the past, with the foci combining object relationship and ego psychology orientations. On several occasions one or another member of his family was seen, either alone or with the patient. He seemed increasingly self-observant and most ego functions were quite good. The frequency of his drinking markedly diminished, but when he did drink his behavior was often just as explosive and unpredictable as it had been in the past. Drinking episodes often led to activities that reflected at least temporary superego lacunae. Thus, members of his family lived in a state of frequent chaos and anticipatory anxiety.

By this time we had been working individually for about two years, and I was attempting to examine with him the ways in which feelings toward both parents were affecting his relationships with his wife and children. After a particularly involved drinking episode, he stated that he wanted to end the drinking and proposed to do this by being placed on antabuse. He has now been taking antabuse for over 20 years. During the first few years there were several episodes of "dry drunks" in which his drinking behavior was replicated even though he was sober. As time went by, these diminished in frequency and intensity.

The patient continued to be seen for several years after he began to take antabuse. For a time he successfully shifted the focus onto his attempt to remain sober, and the focus shifted further with the difficult and terminal illness of his wife. Subsequent to her death he terminated treatment but continued to come in from time to time for consultation in reference to childrearing problems (now adult, some of the children have done well, but one has had a criminal career and another is a polydrug abuser), then later with respect to his remarriage.

Now almost 70 years old, he is part owner and vice-president of a small publishing company. His second marriage may be described as friendly and relatively tranquil. Contact with those children who are nearby ranges from casual to relatively close and is accompanied by a quiet yearning cloaked by some attempts to minimize the extent of his desire. In 1988, after a hiatus of somewhat over two years, vigorous, and still on antabuse, he saw me for several sessions. He was frightened as a result of having suffered several small strokes. We talked of his recent life, his worries, plans, and prospects. There was a bit of reminiscing, then later a call to say he was doing better. Perhaps I shall hear from him or about him again.

What shall be said about this man and his treatment? Was it only a symptom cure? Was it even a symptom cure? After all, he had to continue, or in any event felt that he had to continue, to take antabuse. Might it have been more than a symptom cure? Subsequent to the intense period of his treatment, he weathered many hardships and, in distinction from earlier times in his life, was able to more accurately gauge difficulties early and, on his own initiative, seek therapy, which he then used well. Further, he gradually developed a life that had its own warmth and was as rewarding as many. Yet it seemed that he never quite grappled with his relationship with and feelings toward his parents to the extent I thought he might. Was it what Eissler[1] would have characterized as a flight into health? Or had he grappled with it subsequently, in his own time, more than I knew? And yet again, might his subsequent progress have been accounted for simply by the passage of time? It would be hard to demonstrate definitively, but my observation of other alcoholics over the years makes this last possibility seem quite unlikely.

Then there is the question of the dry drunks and the antabuse. What does this say about the psychology and physiology of it all? With respect to the dry drunks, to what extent might the drinking have been a mask for bipolar or other disorder? What might be said of his staying on the antabuse all this time, and what ethical questions would have been involved in attempting to take him off antabuse?

Questions that I would like to have dealt with—the choice of or interplay between hospital groups, individual therapy, medication, work with families and employers of alcoholics—require examination and discussion elsewhere. Here it is sufficient to note that the orientation should be kindred to that which I conveyed with respect to work with Alcoholics Anonymous: The determination should not be made by fiat but on the basis of psychodynamic assessment of the particular patient, his or her situation and needs, the quality of the patient's environment, and the strengths and limitations of the resources available.

In this paper, approaches to the treatment of alcoholics have spanned a number of loci of intervention and treatment modes, including some that may seem cognitive, behavioral, and pharmacological. What relation has this to anything psychoanalytic? A number of factors make this psychoanalytically oriented psychotherapy, and these have been alluded to throughout the paper. The view of the person, of people's development, of their organization, and of the world in which all of this is embedded is psychoanalytic. The need for individual and specific diagnosis, and the treatment based upon this, and, finally, the assessment of the relationship between the patient and therapist and the determinants of the crucial interactions between them is psychoanalytic. Clearly certain principles apply that, not so strangely, apply as well to work with people having other emotional difficulties: In general when work begins earlier, there is a greater possibility of success; if the person having the difficulty begins to hurt—in distinction from inflicting hurt upon others—there can be a greater possibility of success.

Sigmund Freud (1927) said, "The voice of the intellect is a soft one, but it does not rest until it has gained a hearing." In work with alcoholics, the therapist's voice, which must be that of a disciplined and compassionate intellect, must so engage the patient that he or she will hear, will remain, and will join his or her voice with the therapist's again and again so that they can effectively accomplish enough of what they have set out to do.

Notes

1. Eissler, K. R. Paper presented in Chicago.

References

Freud, S. (1921). Group psychology and the analysis of the ego. *Standard Edition*, *18*, 67–143. London: Hogarth Press, 1955.

Freud, S. (1927). The future of an illusion. *Standard Edition, 1*, 3–56. London: Hogarth Press, 1955.

Parsons, T. (1964). Definitions of health and illness in the light of American values and social structure. In *Social structure and personality*. London: Free Press.

Schechter, D. E. (1959). The integration of group therapy with individual psychoanalysis. In *Psychiatry: Journal for the Study of Interpersonal Process*, *22*(3).

Sheahan, J. (1979). *Essential psychiatry*. London: MTP Press.

Chemical Dependency and the Denial of the Need for Intimacy

Arthur S. Liebeskind, M.D.

In psychological terms, the severest blow of chronic addiction falls on the need for intimacy, on the need for people as primary sources of human satisfaction. When one talks about intimacy culturally, one talks about such experience as falling in love, having someone become significant to you and vice versa, having someone to share your most private thoughts and feelings. What we find in the chronically addicted is a severe denial of this need for intimacy. The addict actively repudiates the need. The need for intimacy is disowned, and if it reappears or threatens to, it is met with horror, disgust, or total alienation. In the chronically addicted population, we see no relationships or relationships based on mutual distance, driven by the classic dynamics of distancing operations. Chronic addiction leads to progressively non-intimate relationships.

Psychologically, the original experience of intimacy occurs between the infant and the mothering one (Sullivan, 1953). Note it is the mothering one, not the biological mother. The mothering one can be an older sister, an aunt, a father, a grandmother, etc. It is the person who cared that the infant survived and therefore gave it some tenderness and responded to its needs. Moving on to childhood, ages 2½ to 4, tenderness occurs with a range of other adults as well as in the parallel play interaction with children of the same age. In the juvenile period, ages 4 to 8, intimacy is extended to experiences of cooperating, compromising, and non-hostile competition with peers, all with the accepting validation of the parenting ones. During preadolescence, ages 8 to 11, intimacy is further enhanced in love between friends, wherein the peers' needs become as important as one's own. In adolescence, this intimacy continues in developing friendships and, with the addition of the maturing sexual need, finds new ground in erotic love relationships (Sullivan, 1953).

Chronically chemically dependent patients appear to be fixated in the infancy mode of the need for intimacy. As will be elaborated later, chronic addiction is viewed as a deterioration in the capacity for intimacy. This can occur in any person from whatever level of interpersonal competence they had achieved. An individual who has deteriorated in a major way ends up fixated in infancy.

At this stage the person feels a need for the original mothering that he or she never had. Fantasies are typically fixed on the mother/infant experience. A person fixated in infancy is also likely to perceive others, including the therapist, as an authority engaged in power plays, or may perceive him- or herself power oriented, needing to impose his or her authority on others. The perception of authority can be all good or all bad and can shift momentarily. The individual at this stage perceives a potential parallel play situation (like a group or a meeting) as authority dominated and therefore filled with danger, such as of being attacked, criticized, overpowered, manipulated, dominated, driven crazy, etc. The parallel play situation is not experienced as a comfortable, potentially exciting group experience with peers who enliven one's life.

An addicted individual lusts after, craves after, the drug or alcohol, not the person, relationship, better working condition, or better education—all that productive ambition would lead to. Addiction eliminates long-term goals. What the addict wishes for is momentary—a fix, sex, a thing, a car, a trip, an orgy, a different sexual experience, a different subjective, chemically induced mood experience that is intriguing or relieves a dysphoric state.

Theoretical Overview

An extensive overview of theory can be found in Khantzian and Shaffer (1981). They review many different motivations for addiction: pleasure seeking (Rado, 1957); tension relief (Fenichel, 1945; Savit, 1954, 1963; Wieder & Kaplan, 1969); defense against aggression and sadism (Glover, 1956); avoidance of mastering developmental conflicts (Hartmann, 1969); and substitution for defects in ego defenses (Khantzian, 1972); Wurmser, 1972). They also note the influence of conditioning (Wikler, 1965).

Levin (1987), influenced by Kohut, emphasizes the regression to pathological narcissism, depriving the ego of its object and activity bonds. Levin reviews object relation theorists, like Kernberg, who see parallels between psychic mechanisms in alcoholics and narcissistic personality.

Zinberg (1975) theorizes that the addict's increasing dependence on the environment impairs the ego's autonomy from the id, which impairs the ego's ability to relate to "objective" reality. Zinberg and I agree that addiction is a function of a particular person living in a particular culture/subculture, at a given time, with a certain availability of drugs, rather than a function of a particular psychopathological character structure.

It is hard to equate Sullivan's (1953) "self system" with the psychoanalytic "ego"; Sullivan refers to them as cousins or closer. Pearce and Newton (1963) divide the self system into productive and restrictive parts. The restrictive part is organized to restrict functioning in the service of restricting intimacy. In this paper, deterioration can be viewed as a further streamlining of the self system to its restrictive part.

Study

When patient life histories were reviewed in an outpatient, inner city, mental health clinic and methadone unit, patient's history of important relationships was typically relegated to an unimportant and totally separate existence from the world of the drug life. Significant relationships and awareness of them simply were not the crux and stuff of what gave meaning to the addict's life. The individual tells you what his or her priorities are. They are usually the crises, the external emergencies, the details of the drug life. One has to ferret out that the crisis is often interpersonal—a loss, a separation, a death.

The economy of scarcity is the addict's orientation to intimate relationships. Life is based on the premise that there is emotionally only very little to go around, and therefore little is all one can expect.

Let me expand. When I examined the life histories of the chronically addicted, particular themes emerged: There was at least one love affair, there was one good job, there was one family experience with children—and then there were none. There was never a repeat. The person was knocked down and never got up for the second round. In the belief system of these people exists the idea that they had only one chance. If they failed, life was over; they became committed failures. The failure was proof that the individual was not capable of aspiring to anything better; the one chance was used up.

Particularly in the poor and lower class population, where abuse, abandonment, rejection, and deprivation are often the stuff of childhood, taking a chance on another human being is a remarkable event in itself. It is the high point of life. When patients talk about it, their eyes light up, or they get grim with rage and hurt. Sometimes even taking this chance had the seeds of its own sabotage already in it, for example, the young teenage couple, madly in love, but both heavily into the drug life.

When I talk about experiences of love, I use the term relative to the individual. It was the point in life that the person, if only for a moment, trusted, shared, felt excited with another human being, could talk about him- or herself to the other, could feel someone cared whether he or she lived or died. This was a point where humanness was the priority. In some, the humanness existed mostly in fantasy, but the object was a real person. Often drug taking at the time was perceived as facilitating the relationship.

For others, it was a group that provided the experience of intimacy. One patient reported that the first people who cared about her were those in an adolescent group who taught her how to survive. But whether it was an individual or a group, the experience of intimacy made the person feel more open, assertive, sexy, witty, attractive, in short, more able to survive in a dangerous world. Often this point is very buried. It takes an investigator some time to uncover it, and the moment of hope that went with it.

After the disruption of the relationship, a morbid preoccupation with the failure may roll around over and over again in the individual's consciousness. For some, it is the secret that they never want the therapist to know, for example, the day they left their children to an uncertain fate, the day they drove the woman they loved out of the house, the time when life was going so well they took the family savings and blew it on drugs. For some the remorse about this secret is still a hot issue, 3, 5, 10, 20 years later. For others the memory of the lost experience is buried. The hurt is so great that the patient dissociates it and, so to speak, lives out the life of the person who is doing penance. One patient reported never talking to anyone about the one woman he loved whom he lost because of drugs. He wanted from me some confirmation that his problem was a chemical imbalance, a symbolic statement that he never should have become involved with people in the first place and should resign himself to do without people in the future. Another patient, after four years of psychotherapy, revealed that she did love one man. He married her when she was 18, and saved her from her abusive family. He died suddenly in an accident, and in her remorse she became addicted for the next 20 years.

For others, there is a frank denial that a love experience ever existed or, if it did, that it had any significance whatsoever.

The morbid preoccupation with failure becomes the obsession that stands in the way of any future changes for the better. What goes wrong is not that the individual had a significant relationship that failed, but that he or she became afraid and did not try it again. The avoidance of future attempts is rationalized in many ways. Examples are:

"She was a saint. I was a bastard for what I did to her. Bastards don't deserve anything."

"That relationship was a disaster. After a while she led me on. I followed. She never delivered. Who needs disasters? It was a mistake to have taken a chance on love. So I'll be lonely. Who cares?"

"Yeah I loved him. But in a little while, I got pregnant, again and again. He kept me home that way, so he could go out and I couldn't. It was a way of putting me in prison. No, never again. I ain't going to let any man put me in prison again."

Chronic addiction is a problem of deterioration. In the chronically addicted we observe the process of deterioration from a high point or points of intimacy. The highest point of intimacy an individual has achieved might be the adolescent group that provided the substitute family. Deterioration is both psychological and (often) physical. The ultimate effect of all these processes is the writing off of the need for intimacy. Some of the processes involved are:

1) Projection of blame to the outside and the subsequent increased derogation of others.

2) Retrospective reformulation of the events of one's life, which has the effect of excluding by omission or change any memory of a person who was a source of tenderness. This retrospective reformulation can also eventuate in an idealization of the destructive people in one's life. The idealization can range from one's non-nurturing mother to an enabler to the entire destructive drug culture.

3) Progressive isolation from others and denigration of the meaning and importance of relationships.

4) Progressive taking of increased risks with one's life. How often do we see patients who ignore minor ailments and allow them to become major diseases. At best, self-care is of a band-aid nature.

5) Progressive decrease in the fantasy that a good mother type person will appear. The addict even loses the hope of this idealized fantasy. This, in turn, leads to even fewer expectations and fewer goals. Less is expected from a therapist and the therapeutic experience, and cynicism and despair reign.

6) Progressive tolerance for and use of drugs to deal with any and all moods and states of being. The drug is more and more perceived to be the external controlling agent of mood.

7) Streamlining of one's interpersonal orientation to others. Whereas before, the individual could see that one might have to be civil to others to get what one wants, or could agree that it was in one's best interest to go to work and be responsible, with chronic addiction, all the self-centered orientations come to the foreground (the personality disorders). For example, the addict feels routinely entitled to this or that, or is narcissistically demanding or all dependent on this one or that one. The self-centered orientations can represent a deterioration from the time when the individual thought that human relationships, in and of themselves, had some intrinsic value. Now the thought is "whatever you do for me is too little, too late, useless, not enough, too inconsiderate, rejecting, etc."

8) Progressive restriction in the range of emotion with a progressive increase in anger. The anger may be repressed so that the patient presents him- or herself as emotionally flat. That same patient can have rages, but the basic emotional range is flat. Neither sadness or joy are experienced. These emotions represent a more direct caring connection with others.

9) Progressive loss of function. For example, after many years on drugs, the patient who once worked, played sports, danced, talked, and lusted after others cannot pursue or perform any of these functions in the present, or does so with great difficulty.

10) As the content of consciousness becomes more and more restricted, and expressiveness become limited, communication becomes more organized to deceive, to control, and to frighten, rather than to express an honest thought or feeling. In fact, language itself becomes more narrowed, filled with more aggressive words and intonation.

There is also deterioration that sometimes follows a psychotic episode. Such deterioration involves increasing paranoia and further isolation. Many of our dual-diagnosis patients fit into that category. However, often the paranoia may not be clinically diagnosable, as in ideas of reference or delusions, but shows up in more subtle ways, such as a chronic distrust of people. Our patients engage in the drug culture, where the unspoken agreement is "never let yourself be put in a position of vulnerability."

What helped me to relate chronic substance abuse/addiction to the denial of need, and specifically the denial of the need for intimacy, was my experience in the sixties on the detoxification ward at Metropolitan Hospital. Young addicts during the process of withdrawal from heroin described a number of personal events: They became hungry; they began to feel lust; they became aware of colors and sounds, sometimes to a frightening degree of intensity. They began to dream, some with frightening nightmares. This was not only their subjective experience, but they were observed by the nursing staff to change in a few days of hospitalization from being toned down to being emotionally labile. Overt rage, jitteriness, having a short fuse, increased hunger, and sexual desire were all observed. It was as if a great veil, a great weight, had been lifted. Emotional life had a greater range, the experience of desire was liberated. What Sullivan (1953) described as "uncanny emotion" was often experienced, along with desire, loathing, terror, panic, rage, impending doom. The emergence of these emotions, no longer held in check by the effect of the heroin, was often enough to propel the person precipitously and prematurely back into the street and onto drugs. Often a repressed suicidal impulse came to consciousness and the patient signed out only to kill him- or herself.

What I and others observed was the lifting of the suppressant and dissociating effects of the drug on the adult personality. What emerged was intense desire, intense longing, intense emotion, and often intense despair. The dreams I collected were filled with horror images. Some spelled out symbolically the bases of the logic of why intimacy should not be a part of one's life, but denied. One dream comes to mind. The patient reported that he was shooting up. The syringe was in his vein. He pushed the drug in his vein, but soon the blood began to push back and go out the syringe into a tube that was attached to the end. He followed the tube out of the room into the hall. In the hall was his mother with the tube in her mouth drinking his blood. The connection with heroin was equated with the connection to his mother, the original model of the availability of tenderness.

What was seen in the detoxification ward was the needs and emotions that were dissociated/suppressed in the patient during addiction, and the logic of what recommended their deterioration. In detox, the gap between needs that once were thought capable of being satisfied, and what had actually happened through the current life and consciousness, was experienced. The perceived abyss between what the patient once thought was possible in some context of intimacy and what the patient had done with his/her life while on drugs was often enough to drive the patient back to drugs, or to suicide. During detox, the security operations of the self system (ego defenses) had temporarily not operated as efficiently, allowing the dissociated/suppressed to come through into consciousness.

Was the patient first pathologic or did he or she become pathologic after the chronic use of drugs? It is both. Drugs are used to service the pathology, to make it operate smoother, and drugs create pathological states. Everyone has his or her own way of dealing with anxiety and depression. By the time one is in adolescence, one has an efficient distancing system from people. This antianxiety system is maintained by distancing maneuvers that try to prevent blows to self-esteem. The more unsuccessful a person's life experience is vis-à-vis people, the greater the necessity is to distance from people. Without intervention, the natural result of a series of negative interpersonal relationships is cynicism. Distance operations increasingly dominate in the adult personality. One gets lonelier and lonelier, yet one denies one's need for people. As the loneliness becomes increasingly painful, it gets more dissociated or suppressed.

Now drugs come on the scene. Depending on the individual and his or her predominant mode of security operations or distancing maneuvers, a given drug treats the pain that results from deprivation of needs, particularly the chronic denial of the need for intimacy. Dysphoric moods are made to feel better by the drug. But that is only fleeting. More dysphoric moods are produced. So these are also medicated. The availability of drugs allow a person to medicate in any direction—up, down, etc. The more life gets devoted to drugs, the more the focus is away from the human field, and the loneliness grows more intense. The distancing from people gets more severe, which creates more and more loneliness, as the cycle goes on. Often the experience of loneliness itself gets dissociated or repressed. More and more dissociation of the need for tenderness occurs.

In dissociation, needs as well as the thoughts and feelings associated with them become pushed out of awareness (Sullivan, 1953). The evidence that they are there, buried, may come out in the form of dreams, or fugue states, or even in the experience of detoxification, as I explained above.

Drugs facilitate deterioration. They oil the distance maneuvers and create new distance maneuvers. Intimacy and the need for it becomes more dissociated. The lifestyle of the addicted person living among addicted people becomes part of the necessary context by which dissociation is maintained. It is not enough to take drugs. One must be with others who are committed to mutual distance to facilitate effectively the denial of the need for intimacy.

Drugs allow the system of the denial of the need for intimacy to work smoother. Drugs tone down rage, make the individual feel less hungry, less lustful, less afraid, less disorganized, less psychotic. Drugs also facilitate role playing and deception, and take the edge off any vestige of conscience that one hurt someone else.

Drugs allow for the compensations of low self-esteem to emerge. With ten bucks for crack, one can feel like a million bucks, on top of the world, the greatest talker, lover, wheeler and dealer, intellect, or friend imaginable. Of course, it last as long as the chemical. In point of fact, drug taking does nothing for low self-esteem except make it lower. Esteem comes from the cumulative successful experiences with intimacy, and all the grandiose plans and intentions the addict has do not do one thing for self-esteem.

When we take a look at the *current* relationships of the chronically addicted what do we find? Interpersonal isolation is common, as are relationships that are purely drug seeking. The mutual agreement is that neither party would ever dare trust the other. The drug comes first. Hanging out with others is motivated by the fact that it feels better than the deadliness of being alone. With some, it is mutual exploitation, with each terrorizing the other in the power game. The best example is the violent blaming so prevalent in addict marriages. Neither partner can break the bond because the terror of isolation is worse than the terror of abuse. The scripts are many, but the basic elements of intimacy are absent. The fear of loneliness outweighs the fear of whatever the other person imposes. A paradox is created. The fear of loneliness drives people to stay together in a state of mutual isolation.

As repudiation of the need for intimacy takes hold, the patient's adult personality becomes streamlined to the pathological, to the distance operations rather than productive functioning.

Crises present a serious problem for the substance abuser. Since maintaining the optimal mood becomes the overriding necessity during crises, the trust of people is sacrificed for the drug need. Paranoia is no longer neurotic in the drug world. One needs to be paranoid to survive. It is justified and necessary, and subjectively it is felt to be natural. Another paradox is created. Unnatural paranoid living becomes the comfortable norm to the paranoid person. Situations of potential trust, like being in the room with a psychotherapist, become filled with danger.

People are chosen who have an equal or greater capacity to avoid intimacy than oneself. The other is as bleakly lonely and committed to the drug world as oneself. In the addict's life, scenarios of betrayals, deceptions, and intimidations are played out with ease. The question of intimacy is never brought up. It just cannot exist.

There is a class of patients who have had a period of success interpersonally and economically. They worked. They lived with someone with whom there was some caring. Then the blow came, often self-inflicted. The decline from that point of success is precipitous. Lives are disrupted, savings accounts vanish, the patient is left without a soul or penny in the world. The despair in these patients is particularly great. Having achieved something and then destroying it is worse than never achieving anything in the first place. The remorse of seeing your life vanish in front of you, by your own doing, becomes a living proof that this is the life you deserve. The memory of what happened before the loss, the memory of the good times, becomes the pain in one's side, a gnawing reminder that needs to be blotted out. In the *Inferno,* Dante says, "There is no greater sorrow than thinking back upon a happy time in misery." What does a formerly successful business man and family man feel, when he, at age 45, lives in a back room of his parent's house as he did at 13, a beggar and a bum to them? This particular dual-diagnosed patient attempts suicide every few months. The resistance against ever trying again is strong.

Therapy

Therapy intercedes in the process of deterioration. We do not have an easy task.

Given that everyone is on the continuum of a process of growth or deterioration, it is important initially to assess the patient's degree of deterioration and degree of hope. Hope, here, indicates the felt need to relate in an intimate way to at least one other person in the real world. The therapeutic relationship is possibly the most hopeful experience the chronically addicted patient can have. That relationship can make the difference between life and death.

Establishing a relationship with a therapist is therefore primary. If the patient is unable to, because of drug use, detoxification is the first order of business. Detox is always the best way to begin if the patient agrees. If not, and contact can be made, therapy can begin without it, but it has to be one of the more urgent immediate goals.

It is difficult to talk about therapy with the chemically dependent patient without seeming trite. All the approaches have some merit and work with properly dedicated and trained personnel. If one accepts the central thesis that the major difficulty is in intimacy and the major resistance is the denial of the need for intimacy, the organization of therapy is clear-cut. The goal for the patient has to be to revive the need for people. The goal of the therapist is to formulate the problem and direct therapy toward the patient's need to be with and relate to people, not people who are abusing substances, but people unencumbered by such problems.

Psychotherapeutic Considerations

The therapist needs to fit the treatment to the individual patient. Patients who are willing, should detox as the first step. With patients who are not willing to detox, but a connection can occur with the therapist, psychotherapy can proceed. A connection implies the patient's ability to come to sessions, be alert, relate to what is going on, and remember what happens. If the patient is not able, the therapist should consider this absence a serious problem, then work on it.

Patients who refuse to detox, and with whom a connection with the therapist cannot be made, should be advised that they do not wish treatment at this time and should return when they do wish treatment. Working with the family/friends/workplace may be the only leverage to get the patient to act.

In general, the therapist needs to be versatile, ready to insist on detoxification for some, ready to start psychotherapy with others. Once the therapeutic bond is established, the therapist has greater leverage to influence the patient toward detoxification of abstinence.

In psychotherapy, the focus of work typically has to begin with dealing with the character armor. This is where the skill of the therapist lies, for example, in dealing with and confronting lateness, missed sessions, absence/obscuring/distortion of communication, intimidation, deception, etc. Here the goal is to help the person become a patient. Confronting these character defenses, with an orientation that defenses had origins to be discovered, typically is something the timid therapist avoids. What can the therapist do?

Very early in therapy, the therapist needs to formulate a life problem for the patient based on as much of the history the therapist can obtain (Sullivan, 1954). The more data obtained from the patient, the more concise and sharp the formulation can be. Frequent summaries need to be given of who the patient is and what the problems with people are.

Sessions should be organized with a focus. If the patient runs with the ball, it is only because the therapist strategically allows it. Insofar as possible, the direction of therapy should be in the hands of the therapist.

Problems with communication are often addressed as one of the first orders of business, for example, "You talk, I listen. Then I talk, and you listen." The therapist should be able to use language the patient can understand—direct, concise, with little or no jargon.

Typically, the patient has a stake in sabotaging therapy. The therapist represents all that the patient has written off, namely, intimacy and the prospect for it. To some patients, the therapist is perceived as the embodiment of the most dangerous threat to their existence (living without the need for people). To others, the therapist is perceived as someone to be manipulated for their personal self-serving, nonintimacy related goals. The patient will do anything, or be anything in a pseudo way, to achieve the self-serving goal. At best is the patient who perceives the therapist as an alleviator of psychic pain, as long as the therapist minds his or her place and is not challenging. Rarely, with chronic addictions, does the patient see his or her problem as intimacy related.

The effect of the patient's sabotaging maneuvers on the emotional and therapeutic posture of the therapist can be devastating or minimal depending on the sophistication of the therapist. The clearer the idea the therapist has as to who the patient really is and where he or she is in life developmentally, the less devastating the patient's sabotaging maneuvers will be. Therapists who get devastated typically are those who preach from their own experience, who do not accurately assess the degree of deterioration and despair in the patient, who wish to perform miracles, and who do not orient to making the patient a patient.

The patient has a great stake in believing intimacy is impossible. The therapist's own orientation to intimacy as something real, inviolable, precious, and lived out in the therapist's own life is the greatest deterrent to all the sabotaging moves in the patient. However, this can erode under the repeated onslaught of a patient's anti-intimacy character defenses, resulting in therapist burnout. Specific factors that contribute to burnout are: the therapist not clarifying that therapy has never gotten off the ground or has come to a standstill so that sessions continue without purpose or focus; the therapist being distracted onto handling solely external crises, so that intimacy problems are not discussed; the therapist getting overly caught up in the drug life and insisting on abstinence; and, primarily, the therapist not focusing on the patient's problems with people as the major source of the patient's difficulties. Therapeutic termination or the possibility of it is usually an underused maneuver to deal with impasses.

Since the patient has generally moved a great deal away from the human field, his or her problems with people can be very obvious. Pathological relationships or nonrelationships in the extreme are common. The therapist, by initially confronting and encouraging the patient to alter interfering character defenses, is, by example, setting the conditions for communication, sharing, respect for data, etc.—all aspects of intimacy. This gives the patient a contrast to his or her intimacy-deficient life.

Setting the stage for therapy typically takes time with the chronically addicted. It is hard work, but not without satisfaction for a determined therapist. However, it is not the fault of the therapist if the patient has made an inner decision to deteriorate. This may be obvious in the beginning or may take time to discern.

Conclusion

My central thesis is that chronic chemical dependency and the denial of the need for intimacy go hand in hand. The denial of the need for intimacy is the central deficit. Whether failure with intimacy sparked the deteriorative process, or the deteriorative process occurred as a result of drug use and intimacy suffered, the need for people remains the core of the problem. As therapists, the one resource that we are expert in and can promote in our patients is free and potentially boundless—the need for people and the need for people to need people. Zeroing in on each of our individual clients and understanding their particular and peculiar problems with intimacy, and delineating a treatment approach based on this evaluation, is what we can do. Therein lies our work and our hope.

References

Fenichel, O. (1945). *The psychoanalytic theory of neuroses.* New York: W. W. Norton.

Glover, E. (1956). On the etiology of drug addiction. In *On the early development of mind.* New York: International Universities Press.

Hartmann, D. (1969). A study of drug taking adolescents. *Psychoanalytic Study of the Child, 24,* 384.

Khantzian, E. J. (1972). A preliminary dynamic formulation of the psychopharmacologic action of methadone. In *Proceedings of the Fourth National Methadone Conference, San Francisco, January 1972.* New York: National Association for the Prevention of Addiction to Narcotics.

Khantzian, E. J. & Shaffer, H. (1981). The contemporary psychoanalytic view of addiction theory and treatment. In J. Lowinson & P. Ruiz (Eds.), *Substance abuse, clinical problems and perspectives* (pp. 465–475). Baltimore/London: Williams & Wilkins.

Levin, J. D. (1987). A self-psychological theory of early sobriety. In *Treatment of alcoholism and other addictions.* Northvale, NJ: Jason Aronson.

Pearce, J., & Newton, S. (1963). *The conditions of human growth.* New York: Citadel Press.

Rado, S. (1957). Narcotic bondage: A general theory of the dependence on narcotic drugs. *American Journal of Psychiatry, 114,* 165.

Savit, R. A. (1954). Extramural psychoanalytic treatment of a case of narcotic addiction. *Journal of the American Psychoanalytic Association, 2,* 494.

Savit, R. A. (1963). Psychoanalytic studies on addiction: Ego structure in narcotic addiction. *Psychoanalytic Quarterly, 32,* 43.

Sullivan, H. S. (1953). *The interpersonal theory of psychiatry.* New York: Norton.

Sullivan, H. S. (1954). *The psychiatric interview.* New York: Norton.

Wieder, H., & Kaplan, E. (1969). Drug use in adolescents. *Psychoanalytic Study of the Child, 24,* 399.

Wikler, A. (1965). Conditioning factors in opiate addiction and relapse. In D. N. Wilner & G. G. Kassenbaum (Eds.), *Narcotics.* New York: McGraw-Hill.

Wurmser, L. (1972). Methadone and the craving for narcotics: Observations of patients on methadone maintenance in psychotherapy. *Proceedings of the Fourth National Conference on Methadone Treatment* (pp. 525–528). New York, National Association for the Prevention of Addiction to Narcotics.

Zinberg, N. E. (1975). Addiction and ego function. *Psychoanalytic Study of the Child.* New Haven: Yale University Press.

Desperate Worship:
A View of Love Addiction

Carol Smaldino, M.S.W.

A close relative of mine died of cancer four years ago. For one solid year he lay in a bed in his home suffering from the cancer which had moved to his spine. The only sunlight he saw in that time was the length and width of a small window, though he lived less than a mile from one of the more beautiful ocean coasts in the world.

In thinking about love addiction, it can be helpful to know that the person addicted may feel afflicted by a dreaded emptiness and dead-endedness, pierced by the light of the vision of the loved one, the wanted one, the one who functions as a window to the world. Even though the window will not bring salvation, it feels like the source of hope, or at least the illusion of hope. And even when one knows it is only an illusion, it can feel better than the pit of nothingness that is its alternative.

This paper presents an understanding and appreciation of the haunting nature of an addiction to love. It appreciates the threat of breakdown revealed by a movement away from the addiction, the potential health in that breakdown, and the possibility for allowing real change. It points to some of our own vulnerabilities as therapists as we make ourselves so very important in facilitating an exodus that offers the only hope for transition from addiction to authentic living. In particular, it explores countertransference in a personal manner, to illustrate some of the sensitivities to this subject all of us might experience in different degrees. And, specifically, it explores the interplay between the dynamics of this therapist and of a particular patient, which highlights the addictive stance in both.

Before addressing some of the psychodynamics of love addiction, it might first be helpful to clarify some of the nuances of the term "addiction." Addiction implies a desperate need, so desperate as to almost blot out a sense of choice. It is not necessarily part of an ideation, as in obsessive thinking, but rather an urgency of perception that the substance craved (in this instance a person) will obliterate the pain which otherwise remains. The urgency remains even when there is some acknowledgment of the substance's inherent flaws and even failure or destructive effects. The urgency of the feelings of need and craving returns again and again to hound and really possess, until the fight is relinquished in favor of surrender, which for the moment can be full of sweetness.

The term "addiction" connotes a craving for something, be it a substance or a person. Within the context of this paper, the emphasis is on transference. In other words, the afflicted party is by no means indiscriminate. The addiction is not a case where "anyone will do." It is rather a situation in which there is a specific transference related to specific personal early history and a dynamic that lends itself to a specific choice of a beloved. For the purposes of this paper, it is important to note that in the choice of addiction, and in the addiction itself, lie attempts to capture or recapture a sense of wholeness and of healing that seem lacking anywhere else. The insistence on an addictive solution can be so extreme as to assume a psychotic proportion in which reality is distorted or almost completely denied, and it can be consuming. At its most extreme, it can dominate all functioning.

It is important also to include here the concept that a person can have a subterranean addiction to a loved one who is not even overtly active in one's present life. It is possible to be married, with children, to have lovers, and still to be dominated by a longing for one's mother or father or other symbolic lover. It is possible for an addiction to be secret, at times even secret from oneself.

A Psychodynamic Understanding: The Large Parent

For the child who becomes prone to a love addiction, the processes facilitating a sense of integrity and wholeness are very much inter-fered with. The steps of growth that pave the way for self-confidence and engagement with the outside world do not unfold but are instead thwarted. It is as though a sense of wonder is not returned by the parent, leaving an emptiness and despair. The wonder, here, is particularly connected to the capacity for self-discovery, personal feelings, and personal capabilities, as well as a general involvement in the world.

But sometimes the parent is wonderful; the parent's arrival is full of wonder. The parent then smiles on the child and the moment is full. The parent in this instant is in great need of being worshipped, and the wonderful arrival may be based on a parent's idiosyncratic readiness or on the parent's awareness of the susceptibility of the child to that worship.

Margaret Mahler has written of the disastrous effect of the mother's unavailability and negative responses during what she terms the "practicing subphase" and the "subphase of rapprochement" (Mahler et al., 1975). In the practicing subphase the child is in love with the world and "seems intoxicated with his own faculties and with the greatness of his own world" (p. 71). It is clear, as we understand Mahler, that the parent can allow and nurture the child's experimenting or induce fear and dread instead of growing confidence.

In the rapprochement subphase, the child's "awareness of separateness grows" (p. 76). The child, aware of the growing separateness, is at times painfully aware. "He must gradually and painfully give up the delusion of his own grandeur" at the same time "he is gradually recognizing his love objects [his parents] are separate individuals with their own personal interests" (p. 79). It becomes clear that the mother has to be committed to the idea of her child's separateness and to her own life and continued chance to develop. If she is not, she may be tempted, as in the case to be presented shortly, to offer a continued sense of grandeur within the sphere of her own omnipotence, thus discouraging the child's branching out on his or her own. The child would continue to look to the mother for a full range of satisfaction and of life instead of learning to see and use the life sources outside the mother.

The child needs the mother's steady interest, her ability and willingness to "playfully reciprocate" (p. 79). If the mother refuses, the child is left paralyzed, beset by panic, without enough neutralized energy to attend to the "evolution of the many ascending functions of the ego" (p. 80). The child is left with a sense of being abandoned and overwhelmed.

It becomes obvious that a crisis in the rapprochement subphase can lead to profound emotional disturbance. It is in this phase that the child's fear of loss of love can be paramount, along with enormous sensitivity to parental approval/disapproval (p. 107), thus leaving a child particularly vulnerable to feeling shamed. The child's autonomous ventures would be inhibited or limited if the experience of being deflated were to become a real expectation.

The outcome of the rapprochement crisis, Mahler states, can interfere with later oedipal development (p. 107). But interestingly, and pertinent to this discussion, she goes on to say that the clinical outcome of the crisis of rapprochement will be "determined by," in part, "the fate of the Oedipus complex" (p. 108). It is the oedipal phase, it would seem, that can seal the proneness to an addictive solution if it, by a combination of seductiveness and rejection, leaves the child, adolescent, or young adult with the yearnings for the magic of a union with the parent in question, while at the same time leaves him or her with a sense of rejection and dejection about his or her objective worth in the world.

Harold Searles (1965), in a highly interesting contribution to an understanding of oedipal love and renunciation, touches on this poignantly. He emphasizes a picture of the child emerging strengthened by the sense that his or her love is reciprocated, even though it is not realizable, because of a larger reality, not for one's own lack of worth. He stresses the ego-enhancing features of oedipal resolution as opposed to a forbidding superego formation (p. 302).

Searles details the extent of damage that can come to the child's ego if the parent, out of a denial of the real passion felt for the child, becomes seductive, then rejecting and disowning. The parent, in such a situation refuses to acknowledge reciprocal love, longings, and loss in the process. Rather the parent "would unwittingly act out his or her repressed desires in the form of unduly seductive behavior toward the child; but then, whenever the parent came close to the recognition of such desires within himself, he would unpredictably start reacting to the child as being unlovable, undesirable" (pp. 302–303). The parent does not want to feel the extent of this passion because acknowledging the passion would lead to acknowledging the necessary relinquishment of that passion, which cannot be consummated or sustained in any near permanent way. If the parent is lacking passion in his or her own life, the loss is particularly agonizing and may even feel tragic, so the parent refuses to be a player in a game crucial for the child.

In this context, Searles continues, the child's Oedipus complex cannot be resolved because "the child stubbornly—and not unnaturally—refuses to accept defeat within these particular family circumstances, where the acceptance of oedipal defeat is tantamount to the acceptance of irrevocable personal worthlessness and unlovability" (p. 303).

The person prone to a love addiction, then, may have the yearning to return to the parent who had the power to bestow and then to withhold the magic of a love that would have blessed and affirmed the child's existence. The craving can be seen as the desperate search for a return to the earlier scene of luxury and despair, the latter making other efforts at love and life colorless in comparison. The parent has remained large then, because the parent has been belittling, by refusing to own the power of the child to evoke feelings of passion, of real importance. Because the parent has been ungiving in terms of facilitating the child's individuation, the child is left with little motivation and confidence in developing coping mechanisms that lead to a growing sense of adequacy.

The person in treatment who suffers from a love addiction stands to experience a sense of disorganization upon acknowledging that the claims of parent love and hope are flimsy and false. The patient is left with a legacy of deep loneliness and aloneness, and finds old feeling states as those of a lost child. The patient is left with the panic and uncertainty that accompany all separation individuation but that are more manageable when the parent is facilitating and stabilizing. The patient is left, if he or she begins to give up the addiction, with the old despair and rages attached to growing, and a deep resentment about actually having to grow up at all. Finally, the patient is left with an actual incompetence, which can feel very disabling and which is the result of having taken a passive rather than active stance over a period of years.

This incompetence is central as we look at the resistances to relinquishing the magical pull of love addiction. The incompetence is the result of passivity being rewarded and attempts at active resolution left unheeded or blatantly sabotaged. In healthy development, the child who needs to recover from a disillusionment over the loss of omnipotence is facilitated in learning methods of coping, methods of resolving conflict in creative and constructive ways. The person "hooked" on a love addiction has frequently renounced more "regular" ways of learning and coping and can be quite undersocialized and inexperienced in effective interpersonal relations. As a result, there is frequently the dichotomy between grandiose expectations and humiliation accompanying any admission of limitation or defeat. The defeats feel global and prohibitive rather than an impetus for exploring new avenues.

In the case illustration that follows, we can see the search backwards, in the patient and as evoked in the therapist, and the struggle to see whether the willingness to experience, among other things, some reciprocal feelings of love and loss might be ultimately life-giving in the present. The elements of love and loss became particularly pertinent as the patient began to grow from a very regressed, starkly dependent, frightened person into a man of substantial promise.

The Case of Joel

Joel is a 39-year-old research scientist raised in a Mediterranean country, who came into treatment when his fights with his wife of seven years were becoming increasingly violent on both sides. From the beginning of his treatment nine years ago, he has been compelling to me as a patient, as he was poignant in his expressions of pain and in his awarenesses, almost Dostoyevsky-like in his intensity.

Joel was the younger of two children and the only boy in his family. His mother was a depressed woman who could at points be warm and seductive. In her mothering, she was often rejecting and cold, particularly at any attempt on Joel's part to do for himself or have a good time. In her early mothering she was seductive and abandoning, giving but withdrawing before relaxed satisfaction could be accomplished.

Joel's father was a mathematician, widely respected in his community and tyrannical with his children. He was demeaning and devaluing of Joel. Joel lived in real fear of his father, which at times was converted into provocative defiance, which would result in a physical beating by his father. Interestingly, Joel's mother, often overtly overprotective of Joel, never protected him from his father's abuse. In fact, she would initiate the request for her husband's disciplinary intervention, often over some mild misdemeanor. Much later in the treatment, it became clear that Joel's mother, seriously threatened by any sign of his separateness from her, would agitate him to some rebelliousness, which would result in his father's final gloomy decree and delivery of punishment.

Joel's father, never an accessible figure of love or support, died suddenly of a heart attack when Joel was nine. His mother, previously capable of stern injunctions, became more docile and at times pitiable in her own demeanor.

Joel never did well in school despite his clear intelligence. He was seen as lazy and recalcitrant and sent to a boarding school for two years when he was 13, where he studied agriculture. He served in the army at 18 and at 21 met the girl who became his wife. Alice, an American from New York, was on vacation at the time of their meeting. She was drawn to Joel's combination of apparent daring and puppy-like qualities. She herself had been deeply hurt and thwarted in her own childhood and saw in Joel a potential soulmate, a savior, and someone who might take from her what she had to give in terms of affection, intellect, and artistic talent, thus validating her sense of her own right to exist.

By the time Joel came into treatment, the marriage had deteriorated to almost constant bickering, accusations, and threats, particularly threats of abandonment. Their little one-year-old girl would witness and become the center of unleashed verbal lashings and laments without any real overt awareness on the part of the adult participants that a child was present. The marriage duplicated Joel's dilemma with his parents: his wish to flee and fly away, his desperate fear of abandonment before his wings were adequate for real independent flight, his fear of retaliatory rage, his recapitulation, his rage on account of his defeated stance, and finally a futile sense of ultimate defeat and impotent rage leading to suicidal despair. The despair would culminate with the lack of hope of taking ownership of his own authentic self and his tendency to see his only alternative as that of a vacant conformity to a will other than his own.

The Treatment of Joel

In the treatment of Joel, the work was always intense because, in part, Joel was frequently flooded, without any real feeling of being centered emotionally. He was the young child who had given up "practicing" in order to maintain a connection with his elusive mother and placate a threatened and threatening father. His spurts of rebelliousness, with his wife or at work, would be followed by a guilty, anxious retreat back to the symbolic parent, ready to be beaten, or beaten already, thus living out a constant reenactment of an unresolved rapprochement crisis. He resembled a prison inmate, or the rebellious protagonist McMurphy in *One Flew Over the Cuckoo's Nest,* fiercely angered over the enslavement in his position but compelled to return, or not to leave at all. Or the child, small suitcase in hand, who threatens to run away, and in extreme cases may really want to do so; but where will he go, as the convincing powers, the ones who could offer him back his self, are at home? At times, even early on, Joel's pervasive sadness seemed to choke him, and his view of life and of his future was full of despair and bleakness.

Although Joel could be charming and quite seductive because of his incisive observations and his physical attractiveness, it was a stature inevitably doomed to crumble. The most striking feature of Joel was the lack of a center, of a continuity of self. He was observant but not capable of incorporating and utilizing the insight, almost as though there were no adhesive holding a piece of putty in place. And he, seeing his own queasiness in the face of life, felt more futile about his existence.

The treatment became, in part, an effort to gradually repair Joel's very damaged ego. He needed a combination of interpretative work and support in the context of a significant degree of attunement, as either support or interpretation alone would have left him without a firm enough anchor. Whenever Joel began to feel more assertive toward his wife, or at work, or in the treatment, he became highly anxious. His role with his wife, as with his mother and father, was that of bad boy, and predictably he would behave in an agitated, provocative way— placing himself in the role of easy target of blame. Although this was a role hateful to Joel, he could reinstate closeness with his parent in this way and avoid the anxiety, guilt, and deep pain of separation.

Since Joel did not always know how or what he felt, he became confused and frustrated easily. The treatment became the vehicle through which to locate Joel's feelings and perceptions, and gradually he began to have some hope of being understood and even making sense. He radiated turbulence, however, and every new development in the treatment brought strong reactions of anxiety, depression, and guilt.

After about four years of treatment, Joel began to experiment with a move toward asserting himself at home and at work. He was beginning to recognize some of his wife, Alice's, responsibility in their fighting, her frequent harshness and dominating style, her own provocativeness. He began, at work, to see himself as more solidly intelligent and looked forward to feeling more sure of himself. It was at this time that he was laid off at work due to economic restrictions and that I went on a maternity leave.

These events, along with a beginning benign experience on Joel's part of the possibility of a future shift into a more mature position in life, were to precipitate a bout of major depression that lasted approximately a year and a half, during which time he did not work and collected disability. The abandonment Joel feared was now reality for him. He felt dead and considered suicide frequently and for longer periods. The breakdown deep within him was reality as well, and this would begin to permit him to begin to build a stronger foundation. (In the period preceding the breakdown, Joel often said that he felt he had no real foundation.)

Being with Joel in the sessions felt like being with someone gravely ill, someone more in death than in life, someone who had been in a concentration camp. I again had to stay attuned and present while sustaining a viewpoint in which life was a real option for Joel. He needed a vast steady supply of hope, which he borrowed before he believed in it, as a small child tries to utilize his mother's conviction that "it will be okay" before he feels it on his own.

Joel's rages, his sorrows, his many tears, and his sense of defeat, pointlessness, and doom were listened to. His wish for, on some levels, fusion with his mother and his yearning to recover her presence and spare her her own depression were dealt with over and over again and have been steady themes throughout.

The power of my asserting Joel's right to live, my capacity to help him, and his capacities for growth gradually spoke to him in a way that seemed strengthening. Joel seemed, in fact, to need to experience the mother who wanted him to live rather than to die, a mother's love that could be strengthening rather than depleting. Like a coma patient who finally moves a limb, he began to show signs of life.

Throughout the treatment, Joel experienced narcissistic injury of a profound nature whenever he felt misunderstood or anticipated rejection. He feared rejection particularly over any show of real independent feeling and feared I would try to dominate him, which led to feelings of hatred toward me. The hatred, in turn, led to massive fears of abandonment, with bouts of panic; this was another theme of continued importance in our work.

Over time Joel was able to share a greater level of emotion, and fantasy, hate and love. He even began to utilize and be receptive to some humor, which, in addition to being a good sign for his future growth, provided some relief to the atmosphere of treatment and made it possible for me to act more naturally. At the slowest of paces, Joel gradually felt greater trust in me and in the process of therapy, which began to mitigate his internal storms and calm the catastrophic reactions that accompanied his any movement.

He began to trust that I would help him grow, though not yet in a way that could be termed consistent. He would, in time, begin to value his own capacities more, and then need to explore the world at his own pace. He left his wife after 15 years of marriage, feeling he was so stifled within the marriage that he really could not grow, and acknowledging his lack of readiness to be in a real sharing relationship.

He began to have more friendly contacts with some people, even a couple of actual friends. He pursued the study of a musical instrument and took courses in acting. He began, slowly, to date a few women, though this was a tremendously conflictual area. The easiest women for him to relate to were women like his mother, sad women who loved his sadness. It was some time before we could effectively start to address Joel's sexuality in the world. The safe women seemed suffocating; any woman attractive to him seemed out of reach. More recently it has become clear that the attractive women represent, in part, the early seductive mother and the threat of his being taunted and then losing his identity to the overpowering woman. But in order to help him in this area, we had to address his willingness to pursue a woman other than me.

In Joel's beginning venturing into the world, he had to do at least two things. He had to neutralize the shame over acknowledging his experienced and real incompetence and inexperience in dealing with practical problems and with people. And he needed to deal with the massive disappointments and fears that accompanied his giving me up as a complete salvation. For Joel, I had come to represent the parent who could save him; he could fly with my wings and be protected from having to develop and use his own. If he never left me, he would never really have to renounce the completeness of the tie to his mother. He would be deprived, also, of having to take his place as a man among men, not as a slave or as an emperor.

Although the treatment with Joel had always been intense, it was at this juncture that my reactions caused me serious difficulty and worry. I had, to some extent, helped to bring him back to life, to "resurrect" him; now it would be time to help him grow, to help him separate from me, to widen his world. He was in love with me, he yearned for a merging, he wanted to be spared his encounter with the past devastation he would encounter again if he really risked moving further away from (symbolically) his mother. He wanted to be spared a passage he feared he was incapable of. He had always, to some extent, sworn loyalty to his mother because she offered him a permanent bed in her home, a permanent retreat from life. She did not offer him a transformed, deepened love that could sustain and nourish him while he might try life on his own. Rather, she offered him the bed, the tea, the merging if he should refuse to pursue his own interests. Here Joel hoped to alter his mother's sequence: He hoped I might propel him, remaining forever in midair with him, forever watching, forever loving and giving. Joel hoped, in essence that we could "have it all," or that at the very least, he could.

Countertransference

Joel's mother had been unable to support and love, or even tolerate, his growing as a separate person, as it would lay bare her own profound abandonment depression. Her own father had been seriously depressed when she was a girl; he had been hospitalized and had shock treatments. Joel became his replacement; she had to try to keep him for herself since her tie to her father had continued to be a major source of longing for her. Alice, interestingly, had a father who was also severely depressed, though at points in her childhood he seemed able to give her something in the way of affection and validation. Joel became, for his mother and wife, a source of salvation. He would, he could, provide the sense of meaning otherwise lacking to them.

For me, in working with Joel, very similar feelings emerged. As Joel began to show signs of life and strength and a more steady intelligence, my own underlying depression and longing surfaced in ways that for a while, were relentlessly disturbing. I was aware of an enormous grief over losing him, as I sensed his emerging in the world with loves outside of me. Searles (1965) speaks of the reciprocal nature of the sense of profound loss when an oedipal victory is given up. But if the loss seems too devastating and the terms too disastrous, the tie cannot be allowed to dismantle. It is held onto tightly, and at times secretly, for fear of another sense of loss too painful to bear.

The loss of Joel, for which I had to prepare in order to help him be in the world, was one I felt unready for. I felt in love with him, and a terrible sadness pursued me with the notion of having to let go of a clinging hope of his saving me. In my own background there had also been a depressed father—appealing, seductive, and then elusive and critical. There had always been a place in my development that lay in waiting, longing for my father's love, longing to revive my father so he might love me. I couldn't afford to see my father's real limitations, as I needed to cling to a notion of his power to save me.

So I hoped to be the princess who, by her kiss, would turn the frog into a prince who would then love her and take her away. In a way, Joel was becoming a prince; in claiming his own resources he was beginning to claim real life, real victory. But it was his life, his victory, not for me to share.

I had a hard time knowing that I had to let go, even though I "knew" it intellectually. I resisted knowing that Joel's love for me was based on transference (Freud, 1915), on my being the mother who would and could help him to grow into himself, and that any real exposure to my needs would flood him, would threaten to destroy him, as did the prematurely and inappropriately stated needs of his mother and then his wife. I had a hard time knowing, too, that my stability was crucial for Joel, that I could not become a true equal, on a personal or sexual level, without sacrificing my real worth for him. I had a hard time knowing, in the trance of inflating Joel's powers, of making him so grand in my mind, that he was so full of profound limitations—no doubt a stance I had taken with my father earlier in life.

I had to somehow rework, then, my own need to give up my magical wishes to merge, to "have it all." I had to relearn, to become convinced, that Joel and I were fated to be separate, not inherently because of unworthiness on either side, but because we each existed within the larger limitations of life. And that within those limitations, exists, really, the only chance for a life energy that is alive and not deadened or strangled.

I had to get ready to accept a level of loss that I had warded off so far. At moments I felt like Joel's mother. Now, in her place, both for her and for me, I had to return to feel the depression, acknowledge it, and begin to feel I might survive it, so that I might let the love in instead of cancelling its power as she had.

I found ways of letting Joel know that losing the prospect of complete love between us was painful to me as well as to him, that it was a loss that was necessary, not on account of his badness, but because of the limitations of us all. It was a humanizing experience, ultimately, because it was a process which we could in some ways share. For me, too, there was a healing in owning the loving aspects of a connection, renegotiating a loss that had been impossible because the love had been banished. Slowly it became clear that Joel, although he had sworn it was me he wanted, was more than satisfied with a growing freedom to belong in life, something he had felt devoid of before.

It seems that in our ways, both Joel and I began tenuously to be grounded in a more reality-bound sense of hopefulness. Searles (1979) writes:

> Any realistic hope—as contrasted to unconscious, denial-based, unrealistic hopefulness—must be grounded in the ability to experience loss. One who has survived the griefs over losses, over disappointments in the past has known what it is for hope to triumph over—to survive—despair. Also he knows that hoped-for changes which the future may bring, no matter how "favorable" or "healthy" (in psychotherapeutic terms) these changes may prove to be, inevitably will bring a concomitant sense of loss in various regards—since, as he knows from his past experiences, the fulfillment of one hope is accompanied by loss feelings stemming from the necessary discarding of the hopes which have been opposing it.
>
> In this same regard, hope comes into being when one discovers that such feelings of disappointment and despair can be shared with a fellow human being—when one discovers, that is, that the sharing of such feelings can foster one's feelings of relatedness with one's fellow human beings, rather than stigmatizing one as something less than human, something alien and unqualified to be included among human beings. (p. 484)

Concluding Remarks

In the case of Joel, it was in many ways the patient who led me to myself. He led me to my longings, my despair, and my own fights against reality, but also to an aspect of my love and to my feelings of love-ability. And he led me to a process of intense grieving, with an emerging hope of tapping certain aspects of my own vitality that were muted before. Joel also made it dangerously apparent how precarious this work can be in areas of hidden vulnerability of the therapist and how tempting it might be for the therapist to refuse access to this pain by perpetuating the addiction.

There are a number of ways in which the therapist might perpetuate an addiction to love. Perhaps the most pertinent, and of concern here, are the subtle ways in which therapists can ward off levels of loss too painful for themselves to bear. The position of therapist is, to some extent, one of caretaker, with many gratifications, which include feelings of importance, adequacy, and worthiness. Patients can be soothing, attentive, and empowering, and their getting healthier and leaving can be threatening to some therapists. But beyond the potential fear of a patient leaving therapy, there can be a subtle but toxic resistance in the therapist against a level of mourning which the love addicted person must reach in order to get better. This mourning involves a deep dependency on and trust in a therapist. It involves a pain that can feel excruciating and crushing to the protagonist but profoundly depleting to the therapist, who not only is a witness but also needs to touch and heal levels of his or her own pain as well.

It can be tempting for the therapist, discouraged by the stubborn clinging to a love-addictive solution, to be overdirective or to become motivated by frustration. The pain the therapist comes to witness may seem relentless. It is similar to that of mourning but the pain does not really diminish in any steady way until mourning can be a convincing alternative (Miller, 1981, p. 43). The pain may quiet down for a while as the patient addicted to a loved one "revives" old hopes and expectations and, in a sense, refuses to die. It can be hard for the patient to be convinced that the only way to a realistic hope of any semblance of wholeness is to kill off that power of seduction, particularly when real individuation has lost its appeal in a person's life. Real love, or real wholeness, can seem like a meager prospect when compared with the enchantment of worship and the sense of endlessness and timelessness that sometimes accompany that worship. The therapist who contributes to the patient's shame rather than self-respect can be devastating and can duplicate the parents' provocation of the patient's retreat from, rather than entry into, life.

The therapist can feel frightened of the dependency necessary for the patient to be able to confront a depth of inner emptiness, and might push the patient back to the addiction or to other outside sources. The therapist might be too frightened of the degree of emptiness and of grief to sufficiently "hold" the patient in times of great upheaval, and might try to distract the patient away from material necessary for real growth, for frequently the patient who is in a love addiction may look more ill and debilitated when turning points are approached.

Finally, as has become implicit in this discussion, there is the inherent danger of the therapy switching the source of addiction but not loosening the dynamics of the addiction itself. As psychotherapists, we are loved more than most, and often become the center of focus in patients' lives. Even when being actively hated or assaulted, we can still be gratified by the importance we hold. There are therapists in need of worship to the extent that they cannot allow the disillusionment that might really free a patient from deep conflicts and ultimately from the therapist.

No one in the grip of an addiction to love assents to the losses inherent in giving up the addiction without a fight, and that fight will hopefully find its way into the treatment room. Hopefully in the treatment, the affects of this fight can be tolerated and respected.

The early despair associated with the failures at true separateness to convert itself into safety, availability, loving, and taking risks in the real world is a profound and radical passage. It is for the therapist to witness, to facilitate, and to a greater or lesser extent to experience or reexperience a dying of certain aspects and a rebirth as a more separate being. It is to try to pick up the pieces of a broken past and to grieve over what we may not have had—the love we truly needed like oxygen—and what we can never have—the absolute fulfillment with any other human being.

References

Freud, S. (1915). Further recommendations in the technique of psychoanalysis: Observation of transference—love. *Collected Papers* (Vol. 2, pp. 377–391). New York: Basic Books, 1959.

Mahler, M. S., Pine, F., & Bergman, A. (1975). *The psychological birth of the human infant.* New York: Basic Books.

Miller, A. (1981). *Prisoners of childhood: The drama of the gifted child and the search for the true self.* New York: Basic Books.

Searles, H. F. (1965). Oedipal love in the countertransference. In *Collected papers on schizophrenia and related subjects* (pp. 284–303). New York: International Universities Press.

Searles, H. F. (1979). The development of mature hope in the patient-therapist relationship. In *Countertransference and related subjects.* New York: International Universities Press.

Bulimia: A Self Psychological Study

Eleanor Bartholomae Liebowitz, Ph.D.

Some psychological studies discuss anorexia nervosa and bulimia as two sides of the same illness or as sister illnesses (Welbourne & Purgold). There are times when the anorectic exhibits bulimic symptomatology—the binging and vomiting, the stealth with which the food is eaten. Conversely, there are bulimics who try to starve themselves. Even though few of these ever starve themselves so as to send their weight plummeting below normal, their behavior, thought patterns, and psychological disturbances exhibit similarities to those of the anorectic (Welbourne & Purgold). Both have problems with issues of control, dependency, autonomy, and separation/individuation. However, the patients I have worked with have not exhibited the anorectic behavior of starving nor the thought pattern of wishing to be bone thin and seeing themselves as fat when they are not. In addition, they have maintained normal body weight. While this is understandable during binging and purging, the weight has been maintained years after the binging and purging have stopped. Since I have not worked with anyone exhibiting the starvation aspects of anorexia nor the body distortion vis-à-vis slimness, I limit my discussion to that of bulimia. Nor is it within the scope of this paper to discuss whether anorexia and bulimia are two sides of the same illness, sister illnesses, or separate illnesses.

I do believe, however, that the person with bulimic symptomatology is suffering from an addictive disorder. I say this because my patients were compelled to overeat, to gorge, and then to purge. Not one of my patients, during her compulsive behavior, could eat three normal-size meals a day, but had, in seclusion, to put away enormous amounts of food. There was no control over the amounts eaten; the need to eat was a driving force. The food was never enjoyed; its ingestion and purgation were needed to momentarily feel good or to quell anxiety, depression, or an inner feeling of emptiness. I am not implying that my patients were aware of these feelings. Two were conscious of a terrible urgency. One felt a void that had to be filled. The anxiety and/or depression and/or emptiness emerged as the self grew stronger and the need to binge and purge lessened. Although bulimia is not, as far as I know, generally recognized as an addictive behavior, Bemis (1985) views it as addictive, writing,

> Bulimia may meet criteria for addictive disorders . . . in that it involved
> a) loss of control
> b) preoccupation with the abused substance
> c) use of the substance to cope with stress and negative feelings
> d) secrecy about behavior
> e) maintenance of addictive behavior despite aversive consequences.
> (pp. 407–437)

Also, Neuman and Halvorson (1983) write that "Dr. Arthur Crisp of England sees binge-eating as an addiction . . . a carbohydrate addiction requiring ever increasing amounts of carbohydrates and resulting in both physical and psychological dependence" (p. 56). They add that "Gretchen Goff of the University of Minnesota's Outpatient Psychiatry Department proposes that bulimia be viewed as an obsessive fear of fatness combined with an addiction to food" (p. 56).

Kohut (1977) writes that behind the addiction is the structural void that the addict is trying to fill.

> It is the lack of self-esteem of the unmirrored self, the uncertainty about the very existence of the self, the dreadful feeling of the fragmentation of the self that the addict tries to counteract by his addictive behavior. (p. 197, footnote)

While other studies have discussed the emotionally deprived background that gives rise to the symptoms of bulimia and the treatment needed to end the disorder (Bruch, 1973; Cauwels, 1983; Sugarman & Kurash, 1982; Swift & Letven, 1984), this study will focus on a self psy-

chological approach to the dynamics and treatment of bulimia (cf. Barth
& Wurman, 1986; Goodsit, 1983).

I use this approach because addictive behavior, as Kohut (1977)
asserts, is the outcome of deficits within the self. Over the years, I have
learned that my bulimic patients suffer from deficits in their self-
structure brought about by empathic failures in their lives. In the
upbringing of my patients, the phase-adequate mirroring, idealization
processes, and deidealization processes that would have allowed for
the structure-building transmuting internalizations to take place did
not occur.

> When a "tolerable" phase-appropriate loss of some discrete
> function that the object carried out for the child is experienced
> ("optimal frustration"), the psyche does not resign itself to the
> loss; instead, it preserves the function of the object by internal-
> ization. When "effective internalization" replaces a function of
> the auxiliary ego by an internal structure that carries out the same
> function, a process has taken place that can be described as a
> structural "leap." For example, what the mother does for the baby
> when she rocks him to sleep, or later for the toddler when she
> reads him a story, is eventually replaced by a structure that
> enables the child to go to sleep by himself. This "leap" is ac-
> complished by transmuting internalization, an intrapsychic
> process that involves "a depersonalizing . . . of the object, mainly
> in the form of a shift . . . from the total human context of the
> personality of the object to certain of its specific functions" . . . .
> Thus, when the narcissistic object cathexes are withdrawn
> ("abandoned") from the lost function of the object imago because
> of optimal frustration, the object's function is preserved ("pre-
> cipitated") as "a particle of inner psychological structure that
> now performs the functions which the object used to perform
> for the child" . . . . (Tolpin, 1971, pp. 317–318)

The primary goal then of treatment is to strengthen the weakened
self-structure. Through the use of empathic mirroring, by providing a
milieu in which idealization and deidealization processes can occur,
transmuting internalizations take place and the necessary structuralization occurs. An approach, therefore, that would focus on intrapsychic
conflict, on exploring and analyzing defense mechanisms and resistances, or on interpreting drives does not allow for transmuting
internalizations and therefore does not strengthen self-structure. And
because such an approach bypasses the patient's "subjective internal

experience" (Magid, 1984, p. 102), it causes these patients to feel misunderstood and at times attacked.

I have found that empathic resonance with my bulimic patients' defenses, resistances, and perceptions of their world and of me, no matter how distorted the perceptions, not only helps strengthen self-structure, but often brings forth genetic material. Moreover, it has been my experience that when self-structure becomes stronger, the patients' perceptions become more realistic, the need for pathological defenses weakens, and the underlying motives and meanings of the defenses and resistances can be explored and analyzed.

In writing of drug addiction, Kohut (1971) states:

> In the realm of narcissism very early traumatic disturbances in the relationship to the archaic idealized self-object and, especially, traumatic disappointments in it may broadly interfere with the development of the basic capacity of the psyche to maintain, on its own, the narcissistic equilibrium of the personality (or to re-establish it after it has been disturbed). Such is, for example the case in personalities who become addicts. The trauma which they suffered is most frequently the severe disappointment in a mother who, because of her defective empathy with the child's needs (or for other reasons), did not appropriately fulfill the functions (as a stimulus barrier; as an optimal provider of needed stimuli; as a supplier of tension-relieving gratification, etc.) which the mature psychic apparatus should later be able to perform (or initiate) predominantly on its own. Traumatic disappointments suffered during these archaic stages of the development of the idealized self-object deprive the child of the gradual internalization of early experiences of being optimally soothed, or of being aided in going to sleep. Such individuals remain thus fixated on aspect of archaic objects and they find them, for example, in the form of drugs. The drug, however, serves not as a substitute for loved or loving objects, or for a relationship with them, but as a replacement for a defect in the psychological structure. (p. 46)

The same applies to food addiction; from the beginning of life "the child asserts his need for a food-giving self-object . . . we might say that the child needs empathically modulated food-giving, not food. If this need remains unfulfilled (to a traumatic degree) then the broader psychological configuration—the joyful experience of being a whole, appropriately responded-to self—disintegrates and the child retreats to a fragment of the larger experiential unit, i.e., to pleasure-seeking oral stimulation . . . or . . . to depressive eating . . . that becomes the crystallization point for the later addiction to food" (Kohut, 1977, p. 81).

My patients suffered from their earliest years and onward the lack of empathic entunement by both parents. There was at best faulty, but for the most part, no mirroring, as well as interference with idealization and deidealization processes (Kohut, 1977). Because of the unempathic self-objects, transmuting internalizations could not take place, leading to structural defects in the self, preventing the ability to self-sooth, preventing frustration tolerance, and preventing the development of self-cohesion and adequate self-esteem (Kohut, 1977). This caused problems in relating to bodily needs, emotional needs, separation/individuation, self-assertion, and self-control. There was a need to use others outside of themselves for self-regulation and particularly, self-esteem. The binging and vomiting provided a momentary sense, albeit pseudo, of cohesiveness and control of life. Conversely, because they needed so much outside approval and, therefore, shaped their behavior to the much needed other, they felt controlled and manipulated. Relations with others were poor, and later object choices continued to mirror the pathological earlier relationship with the parents.

In working with bulimic patients, the reality issues of overeating and purging cannot be the focus of therapy. Food is not the issue. Of course, a defect in self-structure is the underlying issue, but the feelings that arise when the patient begins to search beyond the symptom are anxiety, depression, or terrible emptiness. However, when the patient has the compelling urge to binge and purge, she must do this to quell that urgency.

Only one of my patients felt that the need to binge and purge came from a terrible feeling of emptiness. She ate to fill the void. These patients believe that their lives are not their own. They don't know who they are, what they want, what they feel, what they think. They can only respond in terms of what others want of them.

The greatest pitfall for the therapist is to collude unconsciously in taking controls from the patient. Interpretations, as we know them to be, should be avoided, for the patients are developmentally not ready for them and will use the interpretations, not to make change or gain insight, but to try to figure out what the therapist wants, and behave accordingly. But, even more importantly, as I stated earlier, these patients often feel misunderstood and attacked by interpretation. Given their belief system and behavior toward important others, they turn the feelings against themselves, behaving in accordance with what they think the analyst wants and thereby weakening their already weakened self-structure. In order to promote the much needed structuralization, self-cohesion, and self-esteem, therapists should use interpretations that "focus on, clarify, and acknowledge the subjective internal experience of the patient, rather than those which focus on the distortions in reality brought about by the patient's symptomatology or the transference" (Magid, 1984, p. 102).

Since the patients feel no control over their lives, I believe the therapist, as self-object, has to be flexible enough to allow these patients to control aspects of the treatment situation without interpreting these actions as acting-out or resistances. In the case of my patients, the need to control was exhibited in a need to change the hour of their sessions from time to time. When I could, I allowed for the changes in time and did not interpret. I don't know whether other self psychologists would feel comfortable in doing what I did regarding the changing of hours; nor have I read of this as a self psychological approach to treatment. However, it is my belief that this is necessary, if it arises, in treating bulimic patients. Of course, I am not advocating that the therapist juggle other patients' hours to suit his/her bulimic patients, or to give up his/her own time. But if the time is available, I believe this aids in the treatment. Later on in treatment, when structuralization is more firmly established, this need to control the hours can be explored. Lateness, too, can be a means of asserting control, as can not paying on time. The latter was not used much by my patients, nor was lateness.

Most importantly, the therapist has to be able to accept the binging and purging behavior without interpreting it as a resistance to treatment, and to understand that the behavior has multiple purposes. It is the symptom of the underlying problems in the self. On a more surface level, it is a defense against unacceptable feelings, a means of trying to control an environment over which the patient feels no control, and the only means the patient has to find inner soothing and some momentary semblance of self-cohesion. The behavior is, as yet, the only way that these patients have of expressing inner pain. Bruch's (1973) description of the treatment of anorectics, also applies to the treatment of bulimics:

If the therapist communicates his awareness of the patient's sense of helplessness without insult to the patient's fragile self-esteem, meaningful therapeutic involvement becomes possible, avoiding the exhausting power struggle or futile efforts at persuasion that so often characterize treatment of these patients. (pp. 254–255).

In addition to the above, it is important that the therapist accept the experiential world of the patient as the patient views it and not from the therapist's frame of reference (Stolorow et al., 1987). It is imperative that the world of the treatment situation and the therapists' behavior toward the patient be accepted from the patient's experience of it and not interpreted away as a distortion, as a resistance, or as part of the transference. In other words, the patient's experience of the therapist has to be accepted and validated even though this experience may contain transferential material.* I am not discussing here the real relationship as discussed by Greenson (1978). What I am referring to is a "disjunction" (Stolorow, et al., 1987, p. 162) between the patient's subjective experience of a particular analytic situation or of many analytic situations and the different subjective experience of the analyst of the same situations. When such a disjunction occurs, it is necessary for the analyst to accept the patient's subjective experience and empathically respond to that. Atwood writes of the case of a psychotic woman who kept insisting that her analyst was sending rays out of his eyes that were blocking and piercing her head. The reality, of course, was that there were no rays flooding out of the analyst's eyes. However, this was the patient's inner subjective experience of the analytic situation, and until the analyst realized this and responded to it, there was an impasse in treatment (Stolorow et al., 1987, pp. 161–163).

A less florid example of such a disjunction follows: A patient came into a session and reported a dream. After he told of the dream, he was silent for a while. The analyst asked if he would like to give his associations. He gave them. As far as the analyst was concerned, the

---

* My thanks for this insight to my dear friend and colleague Sandra Jackson. She has had many discussions with me regarding the fact that the analyst can have, without knowing it, an adverse effect on the patient, and must accept this as valid and not interpret it as a distortion or transference. Otherwise we do to the patient what others have done, invalidate his/her perceptions. My thanks for the many conversations Sandra Jackson and I have had regarding self psychology and for all she has taught me.

session ran smoothly; in fact, she felt a great deal of work had been accomplished. The following session, the patient reported another dream. The same sequence followed as before. In the next session, the patient reported a dream, but then told the analyst that her asking for his associations takes the dream away from him and makes it her dream, not his. In trying to explore how this was so, the work fell into a momentary impasse. A transference interpretation not only did not work, the patient felt misunderstood. Not only were his dreams taken away from him, he was misunderstood in trying to tell the analyst about this. When the analyst realized that if the patient experiences that his dreams are being taken away from him when she asks him if he wishes to associate to them, then this is the only reality for the patient and must be accepted empathically, not explored or interpreted away. Once the analyst was able to accept the patient's experience of the situation and validate his feelings, the patient was able to recover the genetic material. His parents had always negated his achievements by asking questions about his achievements rather than by just accepting them. The analyst, in turn, was able to realize that her request for associations had an adverse effect on the patient. And, even though she thought a particular session went well, the patient had a very different experience.

If the therapist responds to the patient empathically, with adequate mirroring, and allows the necessary idealization to flourish and deidealization to occur, a sense of self-cohesion begins to develop and the patient feels understood and begins to experience a sense of control over her life. Self-soothing mechanisms come into play, self-assertive behavior begins, and the binging and purging end. They will reappear from time to time in the treatment situation, but eventually will disappear. When binge episodes are reported, they have to be accepted as necessary and not interpreted as acting-out or trying to destroy the treatment. Even though the symptom may have gone, the work of therapy still needs to be continued so that the self can become securely strengthened.

Hostility, infantilization, intrusiveness, and rigid control by parents were some of the factors present in each household of my patients. These families did not function in empathic entunement to their children's emotional world. They demanded strict obedience and loyalty. The children had no rights of their own. The belief system was that family loyalty was a virtue and mother and father could never be wrong. This belief system could not allow for self-cohesion and inter-fered with the child's developing autonomy, separation, and self-assertiveness. When a child tried to break out of this restricted family structure, she faced the hostility of her parents.

Moreover, there was violence in each of the households, albeit varying degrees of violence. Each of the young women was witness to violent outbreaks by either father or mother, or a father and mother who could not control their rage and screamed and hit and beat when angered or upset. All were witness to the beatings of other siblings, even though they may not have been the subject of the beatings. These parents could not tolerate feelings in their children. Anger was a feeling that was never allowed and was responded to with hostility and sometimes violent repercussions.

The mothers of these patients suffered low self-esteem. They were badly in need of self-objects and used their daughters as such. These women were intrusive, infantilizing, and critical of their daughters. It was difficult for the child to gain approval for anything, be it how she looked, what she wore, her schoolwork, any housework done, her friends. These mothers, so in need of mirroring themselves, could not mirror their daughter's experiential world. They not only continually invalidated the emotional and the reality experiences of their daughters, they needed these same daughters to mirror them to help shore-up their own low self-esteem and fragmenting selves. In order to maintain a sense of self-cohesion, they resorted to screaming, hitting, criticism, or infantilizing. Thus, the development of self-cohesion for the daughters that comes from "adequate empathic mothering could not take place" (Stepansky & Goldberg, 1984, p. 75).

The relationship with the fathers was no better. A significant aspect of the fathers' relationships with their bulimic daughters was that, for the most part, they were absent. One father, after divorcing his wife, no longer wanted to maintain any relationship with his children. He left when my patient was 10 years old and she has not seen him since. He has, over the years, rebuffed all efforts on her part to see him. In the other two cases that I will present below, the fathers were busi-nessmen who devoted most of their time to their job and very little to home life.

However, when they were home, they demanded strict obedience from their daughters, allowing no assertive behavior. For self-cohesion to take place, there has to be not only adequate empathic mothering, but "empathic acceptance of the child's 'voyeuristic' idealization [of the father] and wish for merger" (Stepansky & Goldberg, 1984, p. 75). So if there has not been adequate empathic mirroring from the mother, the child has a second chance for self-cohesion, provided the father can allow idealization, merger, and deidealization, which would allow for transmuting internalizations of the idealized omnipotent self-object (Kohut, 1977). By allowing no assertive behavior, these fathers would not allow their daughters to deidealize them, so there was no way transmuting internalizations could take place.

In addition, both of these fathers denigrated women and openly stated that their sons were more important than their daughters. Despite such statements, the daughters were not allowed to express hurt or angry feelings. The idealized merger with the father had no way of being broken and realistic assessment of him allowed. To add insult to injury, these fathers were possessively jealous of their daughters and were openly hostile whenever their daughters tried to date. Once again, the fathers could not allow for separation. "The presence of a firm self is a precondition for the experience of the Oedipus complex. Unless the child sees himself as a delimited, abiding, independent center of initiative, he is unable to experience the object-instinctual desires that lead to the conflicts and secondary adaptions of the oedipal period" (Kohut, 1977, p. 227). As could be expected, puberty and adolescence for these women were fraught with anxiety.

None of the mothers or fathers got along with each other; fighting was a part of the household climate. The fathers thought of their daughters as auxiliary wives, thereby causing even more anxiety when the daughters tried to date and move out into the world.

I have worked with five bulimic patients in my private practice. I will describe the treatment of three of these patients. All have stopped binging and purging for years now. Two have left treatment and have not binged or purged. One is still in treatment and has not binged for over three-and-a-half years. While all three were able to learn to assert themselves in the outside world, only two were able to confront me when they were upset with me. I do believe that it is very important that the patient learns to confront the therapist when the patient feels misperceived.

Case 1

Hannah, age 23, came to see me after a previous therapist had to terminate treatment. She felt abandoned by the therapist even though she "understood" that after eight months at the agency, therapists move on. She waited a year before contacting me, fearful of losing another therapist. She finally called because she was worried about the binging and purging that had begun again shortly after her treatment ended. Before she would consent to a consultation, she wanted to make sure that I was in private practice so that if she liked working with me she would not have to worry about my leaving an agency.

In the early weeks of treatment, I learned that she had binged and purged on and off from the time she was 18. The binging did not stop fully in her former therapy, but she felt she had received a lot of help and liked the therapist very much. After a while, we increased her sessions to two times a week. Later on, she came three times a week.

She came from a very large family where mother and father worked full time. Mother took time off from work to deliver her babies (there were eight in all, born one to two years apart). She would return to work as soon as possible. Mother had the kind of job that allowed her to be home when needed. However, from the time Hannah was five years old, as the oldest girl, she was responsible for the care of her siblings, both older and younger, when she came home from school. She also helped with the laundry, did the dishes, and, when older, prepared the meals. At age 10, when mother would go on a business trip, Hannah was in charge of running the house. Not only was mother's career more important than the children or the running of the home, father's was as well. He was rarely home, working even on weekends.

No matter what Hannah did to help at home, it was not good enough; mother was never satisfied. Whenever mother was upset with any of the children, she'd tell father. When he came home, no matter how late, he would beat the one or ones that had annoyed mother. He yelled a great deal and had a violent temper. In fact, both parents screamed and yelled often.

Early in treatment, she described her father as wonderful and her mother as a witch. She worried that she could never hope to be the kind of daughter worthy of such a father. He deserved better than her. She was unaware of the discrepancy of her father's yelling and beating her siblings with his being wonderful. While she was the recipient of his beatings only one time, she often saw her brothers beaten. She tried to be a very good girl so as not to arouse the wrath of either parent. She told me that she was never able to finish anything she started. She would begin a project with enthusiasm, which soon abated, and she would then leave the project unfinished. She never graduated from college, for she never completed her final course. She attributed this to the fact that no matter what she did for her mother, if mother found one thing wrong, the whole thing became wrong. Mother would be furious and often made her do over what she had already done.

As a teenager, she began to act-out sexually. She was very much ashamed of this behavior and felt she was no good. Later on in treatment this acting-out was discussed in terms of her search for a caring self-object to get much needed emotional supplies, as a means of trying to strive for her autonomy, of separating, as a means of rebellion against tremendous strictures and controls imposed by her parents, and as the only way she knew of expressing anger.

Her behavior in the early stages of treatment was that of a "good little girl." She was never late, always paid on time, never questioned anything I said, and never expressed any upset with me, even when I took vacations. She always "understood." In working with her, I tried to stay within her experiential framework, accepting her need to be "good," to binge, to purge, never interpreting the reality issues of what the behavior was doing to her body. As time passed, we would discuss her binging and purging in terms of what happened in her life the day of or the day prior to the binge that could have led up to the behavior. As she began to discuss the events of the previous day or the actual day of the binge, it began to become clear that she had been upset over what at the time seemed a trifle. The more she felt accepted by me, the more she could begin to accept her feelings toward those who upset her.

As time went on, the need to binge and purge lessened. At first much self-hatred was expressed as she told me of her binges. I suggested that while we didn't know why she binged, there was good reason for it. This helped to alleviate some of the self-hatred, and she was able to point out the reality issue of the binging and purging being harmful to her body. She eventually came to realize that the self-hatred stemmed from her feelings toward her parents that she did not want to deal with.

While the symptom was growing less intense and imperative, it took about eight or nine months for the binging and purging to stop. However, there were times, for about a year after that, when she would report binging behavior. It was always accepted, never explored, except to ask what had occurred that day. During the time the binging was lessening, she began to be able to explore what it was like to grow up in the household from which she came. We discussed her fears of her femaleness and her feelings of nonacceptance by her father because she was female. Oh yes, he loved her, she was his pet, but because she was female, she was not important. She believed that women are vulnerable to men; men call the shots; women have no control; all they do is work, have babies, and cook. She had no respect for her mother, for she was a career women who allowed herself to be denigrated by father. She recognized mother's intrusiveness into her life. It was ironic that mother was hardly home, yet she was so intrusive, so controlling.

As she was able to verbalize her fear of and anger toward her father, her angry feelings toward her mother were somewhat alleviated. She began to identify somewhat with the mother who, prior to this, had always been unacceptable. She recognized that both parents were never emotionally available to her, and had to allow herself to feel the emptiness and pain that arose. She became aware that she had lived a very lonely life in growing up. She was terribly afraid of being dependent on anyone. In the course of treatment she realized that those fears were because she believed that if she needed someone to be there for her emotionally, to take care of her needs, she would have to give up her self. She became aware of her father's possessiveness and expressed much anger in relation to that.

After two years in treatment, she met and married a man who was as compulsive as she. The marriage had problems almost from the beginning and repeated her early unempathic environment. At the time of the marriage, she began to be late to sessions. I understood the marriage and the coming late to sessions as attempts at trying to separate emotionally from her father and to assert control with me. I did not question the behavior underlying the lateness, rather we discussed it when she brought it up. She saw it as an assertive aspect of herself. She no longer needed to be so "good." She began to confront her mother when annoyed with her, and their relationship improved. She still was unable to confront her father and wondered if she would ever feel approved of by him. She was able to confront her husband. It was during her marriage that she was finally able to confront her father when he upset her, and surprisingly he was able to respond somewhat positively. After three years of marriage, she decided that she would not live in an environment that was not emotionally nurturing for her and began divorce proceedings. She handled the divorce quite well, feeling good about herself.

She left treatment, a year and a half later, having been in treatment with me close to five years, and not having binged for over three years. She was somewhat able to assert herself. I say somewhat, for she was never able to be angry with me, and while I feel that most of the treatment was a success, this part was not. However, at the time she chose to leave treatment, she accepted her femininity and her right to be assertive and to ask for what she wanted. She was able, for the most part, to confront her parents whenever she felt emotionally hurt by them. Her weight was good and her eating habits normal.

Case 2

Ann, age 26, came into treatment to try to control her binging and purging. During her first visit, she told me she hoped we would work well together as she was bulimic and back to binging and purging. She believed that in order not to binge and purge she had to be in therapy for the rest of her life.

The patient, married at 17 to escape a chaotic and horrendous household, had a child at 18, and was divorced at age 20. She began to binge-eat immediately after her divorce and gained 80 pounds that year. She began dieting and lost the 80 pounds. To keep her weight off, she would vomit whenever she would binge, which was quite often. At age 22, frightened of the binge-vomiting cycle, she went into therapy. With the help of her therapist, she stopped binging and was able to maintain normal weight. At age 23, she met a man and entered into a destructive relationship; he was verbally abusive most of the time and at times physically abusive. She was unable to leave the relationship and worked in her therapy to leave it. Prior to seeing me, she did leave the relationship and also the therapist, as he began to treat the ex-boyfriend and Ann felt betrayed, believing that she could not tell him anything about the ex-boyfriend. She began binge-eating and vomiting again when she left treatment.

Ann referred to herself and her siblings as "starving." Food for her filled a void that was too uncomfortable to bear. She also berated the fact that she had to parent her mother, so there was never a real parent for her. She had always felt like "a piece of shit."

As she described her early years, I learned that her parents were always fighting with and screaming at each other and their children. She was second in line of four daughters. Her older sister used to be badly beaten by both mother and father. Ann was determined never to make her parents angry and became the "good little girl" and her mother's confidant, to the point where her other siblings began to reject her. Her parents divorced when she was 10, but even more traumatic than the divorce was the fact that when her father left the mother, he left all of them permanently. He never came back, not even for a visit. He declared that he was through with the entire family. He remarried and moved to another state. All attempts at contact with him by his daughters were rebuffed. To this day, Ann and I are still working with the traumatic effect to her self that this behavior on the part of her father engendered.

At age 12, her mother got working papers for her, and after school she had to work. It was expected that she turn all her money over to her mother. When Ann would ask for some spending money from the money she had earned, she would meet with mother's wrath. When mother was cleaning house, she often would lock her children outside and not let them in, despite their crying.

At age 12, Ann met the boy she later married. She went with him steadily until they married when Ann was 17. She married to get out of the house and away from her mother. However, this relationship recapitulated the earlier one, in that her husband, a child himself, could not give her the emotional support she needed. She had a child at 18, and divorced her husband when she was 20. She began to binge and purge after the divorce. When she was single and dating, she began to realize that her mother competed for her boyfriends. Her mother had always been intrusive in her life, calling daily, demanding daily phone calls, demanding visits, and intruding between the siblings by discussing one with the other.

Mother always admired the children of her friends. She compared her children unfavorably with those of her friends. We can see that there was no empathic entunement for Ann. Her mother, so badly in need of an empathic self-object herself could not validate Ann's experiential world. Since mother could not like anything about herself, which is why her children were compared unfavorably with those of her friends, she could not allow for idealization processes to unfold, and certainly could not allow for the "well-timed process called 'optimal disillusionment'" (Stepansky & Goldberg, 1984, p. 193) to take place. Consequently, Ann suffered and tried to compensate for the structural defects brought about in such an environment. She binged to stop feeling so starved, to quell the void she felt inside. However, the binging and purging was a double-edged sword, for the very behavior that brought some relief from the horrible void brought self-hatred. It was a vicious cycle.

By focusing on what happened during the day of or day prior to a binge, Ann was able to get in touch with the feelings that led to the binge, and the self-hatred over binging began to lessen. As her experiential world was validated in the treatment, she was more and more able to discuss her unhappiness as a child and in growing up without detaching herself from those feelings. The binging and purging stopped after about eight months, and never returned, even sporadically.

We know that for transmuting internalizations to take place which build self-structure, parents must be able to validate their child when he or she challenges their omnipotence and omniscience. Ann's father was unavailable, and her mother certainly was unable to do this. However, the treatment situation can provide the milieu in which transmuting internalizations can take place. The therapist has to be willing to validate the patient's experience of him or her.*

An important example in the case of Ann follows:

In the waiting room of my office, I have a sign that reads: "Thank you for not smoking." Ann was a heavy smoker—two packs a day. Although the binging and purging had not occurred in over three years, she still had compulsive addictive behavior regarding her smoking habit. It seemed to me, however, that Ann had no difficulty in not smoking while in my waiting room and during her sessions. In fact, the year before, I had run a group of which Ann was a part, and for the hour and a half of group, she showed or seemed to show no discomfort about not smoking.

One day, about nine months ago, she came into the office very annoyed with me. (This is a good sign because the patient is asserting herself vis-à-vis the much needed therapist.) She told me she had been annoyed with me since first beginning treatment, but didn't realize it

---

* See footnote, p. 102

until recently. She was a smoker, and an addicted smoker, and I have a sign in my waiting room that, in effect, is telling her that her needs are not important. Since I know that she is addicted to cigarettes, really needs them, suffers without them, what would I do if she were to light up? Would I throw her out, refuse to work with her that day, refuse to work with her altogether? I was tempted to point out the harmful effects of smoking both to the smoker and to me, the recipient of the smoke. This would have invalidated her.

To point out reality would have ignored her needs. Cigarettes were not the issue. What she was asking was whether or not I could put her needs ahead of mine. No one had ever put her needs first. In addition, she needed me to be able to accept her annoyance with me and her disillusionment of me. I needed to accept her intersubjective experience of me as being noncaring about her needs. So I told her that it must have been very difficult for her over the years not to be able to smoke either in my waiting room or office when she needed those cigarettes to feel better. I also agreed that it is difficult to have a therapist who seems uncaring. She agreed that it was difficult at times not to be allowed to smoke and to know that I didn't understand or even care how she suffered during these times. She persisted in asking what I would do if she really needed a cigarette now that I knew how she felt. I told her that her needs were very important. If she felt she needed that cigarette, by all means, she could take one, or two, or the entire pack. She then wanted to know what I would do if the smoke bothered me. My answer was geared to let her know that my needs would not interfere with hers. I did not need her to function as my self-object. I told her that if the smoke bothered me, I'd open the windows, or we would finish the session outside in the backyard. She seemed satisfied and began to discuss other topics. She never did smoke in the office or waiting room.

While this approach to treatment may seem as if I were colluding with Ann's anger and thereby perpetuating her idealization of me, this is not the case. In discussing aggression, Kohut (1977) posits a healthy developmental line that allows for a healthy assertiveness in life. There is also a pathological form of aggression. For Kohut, pathological aggression does not arise due to an innate drive, but is a consequence of a disintegration product caused by the lack of empathic entunement on the part of the self-object.

In discussing difficult patients from the point of view of "aggressions that accompanies a stance from within the subjective experience of the patient and a focus on the more inclusive patient-therapist system as a field of interacting subjectivities," Brandchaft and Stolorow (1984, p. 113) tell us:

> Such excessive aggression is the inevitable, unwitting consequence of a therapeutic approach which insists that certain arrested archaic needs and the archaic states of mind associated with them are in essence pathological defenses against dependency on or hostility toward the analyst. It is the inevitable consequence of the persistent superimposition of the analyst's subjective reality on that of the patient. When this occurs in the treatment, the patient, attempting to revive a previously aborted or derailed developmental step, comes to experience such interpretations, whatever the intent of the interpreter, as severe breaches of trust and as traumatic narcissistic wounds.
>
> A vulnerable patient revives his most personal, nuclear, and vital needs in the relationship to the analyst. When these are misunderstood and misconstrued, and once again the patient is required to see his experiences from another's viewpoint when he so desperately longs for someone to see them from his own, it is not surprising that intense rage, destructiveness, and distrust may follow. (pp. 113–114)

In other words, the analyst must "comprehend the developmental meaning of the patient's archaic states and of the archaic bond that the patient needs to establish with him (pp. 113–114).

In order to provide for the transmuting internalizations that lead to structure building, it was necessary for me not to interpret the anger as a transference reaction, nor to explore the meaning of it, nor to point out, with the view to exploring, the hostility in her behavior, but rather to understand that my patient was trying "to revive a previously aborted developmental step" (Brandchaft & Stolorow, 1984, p. 113) by confronting me about her smoking, by her expression of anger toward me, and by her questioning of whether I would be able to meet her needs rather than mine. By responding as I did, I not only allowed her to revive this previously aborted developmental step, I responded quite differently from the original self-objects. I accepted her feelings and her need to ask that her needs be met.

With regard to whether or not I helped perpetuate her transference idealization of me, let me say a few words about the self psychological approach to the process of idealization. Kohut (1977) has told us that in order for healthy psychic development to take place, there must be "healthy admiration for the idealized self-object" (p. 172). The child searches for the idealized omnipotent self-object with whose power he wants to merge. When this merger is thwarted, self deficits take place. According to Brandchaft and Stolorow (1984), idealization is not viewed as a defense against hostility, but "as a direct continuation of the aborted idealizations of childhood, as a resumption of a tie to an early object which was ruptured by loss or traumatic disappointment" (p. 112). The idealizing by the patient of the analyst, then, is a necessary feature in treatment and will be in effect as long as the patient needs to merge with the analyst's strengths to gain her own.

> The emergence of such an idealization requires no commitment on the part of the analyst to fulfill the patient's archaic expectations, only that the inevitable disappointments be explored non-defensively from the perspective of their current and genetic, conscious and unconscious, subjectively construed contexts. (Brandchaft & Stolorow, 1984, p. 112)

What I did with Ann was to accept nondefensively the fact that she was disappointed in me because, from her subjective frame of reference, I was meeting my needs not hers. Utilizing her subjective frame of reference, I then explored what it meant for her to have me put my needs ahead of hers. I explored from this perspective (putting aside the reality of the situation as I saw it) because that was how the patient experienced the situation. To have done differently would have ignored her subjective experience and repeated what she had experienced throughout her life—the invalidation of her subjective experiences by her self-objects. At this point, no genetic material became available, with the exception that no one had ever put her needs first. Our interaction in this particular session meant that for the first time in her life, she was able to ask that her needs be paramount, and someone heard her, understood, and did not attack. The fact that she could tell me of her anger toward me indicated that deidealization was taking place.

Five weeks after this particular session, Ann came to treatment and told me to congratulate her. She had not smoked a cigarette for almost a week. Instead of smoking, she was trying to get in touch with her feelings whenever she felt the urge for a cigarette. She was beginning to notice that smoking blocked negative feelings. "And, boy," she said, "am I feeling!" She told me she had been asserting herself more at work, at home, with her mother, and with her husband, whom she had married a year earlier; she has gotten him to go to therapy. A few weeks after she gave up smoking, she no longer became entangled in the problems her mother caused between her siblings. Prior to my leaving for vacation, Ann and I began to work on the traumatic events surrounding her father's leaving the family and the feelings engendered because of it.

When I returned from vacation, Ann told me that she was becoming more and more in touch with how much her mother disregards her needs and feelings, and how upset she becomes when her husband or friends invalidate her experiences. She also, for the first time in years, had thoughts of binging. She was frightened by those thoughts and could not figure out where they came from or why they emerged. I asked her if she had any feelings about my being away. She stated that it would have been nicer if I were there, but she understood that I needed a vacation. One of the major problems with the bulimic is she is always ready to *understand* rather than to face her feelings. I told her that I wondered if perhaps the thoughts of binging were related to me and my being away. She told me that if she were angry with me for being away, she was not in touch with the feelings, but she knows that in the past every time she binged it was because she was repressing feelings. I asked her what it would mean for her if she were to discover angry feelings for me. She immediately related that to her fear of being angry with her parents. She blamed herself for her father's leaving, believed that if she had been a better child he would not have left. In addition, whenever she was angry with her mother, her mother would pull away and not speak to her for days, weeks, months, until she apologized for her disrespectful behavior. In other words, for Ann, her angry feelings meant object loss.

In the following session, she told me that while she still didn't feel any anger toward me for being away, she was angry at something I said in the course of the previous session. She explained her experience of me, and once again I empathized and validated her right to feel as she did. Once again, I did not explore, for she needed to know that I could accept her with her anger. As stated earlier, transmuting internalizations result from "optimal frustration." To be annoyed or angry with me for something she perceives I did to her falls into this category. The omnipotent object makes mistakes and is not omnipotent. This all-powerful object can be hurtful, but cannot take offense at hearing that. To repeat, what occurs when the self-object can hear and have respect for the patient's inner subjective experience is that the patient takes in the object's function, and does for herself what the object has done for her. Since I allowed Ann to express her needs, her anger, and her inner subjective experiences, she can now psychically take over my function for herself and allow herself to express her needs, her feelings, her experiences of others, and can expect them to behave as I have done. When they don't do this, she recognizes immediately that she is unhappy with being invalidated.

In the following session, Ann told me that she had an insight. She realized that she "binges on her mother and husband." I asked what that meant. She related that whenever she felt rejected or abandoned or uncared for by them, she would rage and yell, trying to get them to hear her cries, trying to get them to understand, to accept her, to make her feel loved. For her, the insight was that screaming for supplies equals binging, or binging, actual binging, was a scream for nurturing supplies. The following few sessions were devoted to exploring this insight more fully. Two sessions ago, she told me that although life is still difficult, she wakes up every morning with a sense of peace within herself. She loves the feeling.

In the next session, she told me that she is speaking up more for herself than ever before, and doing more for herself without worrying what others might or might not think about her. An example: two co-workers were fighting; one is a good friend of hers. Previously, she would have stayed to bolster the friend's argument for fear that the friend would be annoyed if she did not champion her. Ann wanted no part of the argument and felt her friend was old enough to fend for herself. She walked away and went back to her desk, glad that she was able to do what she felt was best for herself.

During the course of the next session she had a memory return. She told me that on the weekend, her husband walked into their bathroom as she was in there putting on make-up. She panicked and began to yell at him. She could not understand her behavior. She has always panicked at the thought of someone coming into the bathroom after she has gone in there to comb her hair or wash up. In exploring this, she began to cry and suddenly remembered that when she was growing up, whenever her mother was angry with her she would wait until Ann went into the bathroom, then come in behind her, lock the door, and begin to beat her up. Ann could not run away; she was trapped and could not escape until her mother was finished beating her up. Also, in this session, she said that she no longer wanted to be someone else's false image. In exploring the meaning of that remark, she said that her mother uses her children to build up her own ego. Ann no longer wants acceptance based on her being the "good" daughter, the daughter who married well, or the pretty wife. She wants to be accepted for who she is, not for how others see themselves through her. She wants to be loved and accepted when she is angry, upset, depressed, happy, sad. She can no longer be what others want her to be.

Will Ann ever binge again? I doubt it. While she might have feelings of binging, it seems to me that self-cohesion has taken place, the weak self that she came into treatment with has been strengthened. Prior to my writing this, Ann, in her latest session told me that she feels different, her behavior is different from what it formerly was. She said, "You know, I'm finally an adult. I'm in control of my life, and it feels wonderful."

Case 3

Feeling controlled by others is such an issue with the bulimic that the therapist has to be aware from the very first phone call that the patient must be allowed her autonomy. Lee, married, age 23, mother of two, called for an appointment. She had been binging for over a year and was very concerned about it. We made an appointment. Then she asked if I had a few minutes to talk with her. I said yes. She told me that she had just binged on a box of frozen waffles and was feeling very bad about herself. Could I give her advice on how not to binge? I empathized with how she was feeling and told her I believed binging and purging was something she needed to do, even though it made her feel bad about herself. Why she needed to do this was unknown to both of us. I asked if she would like to tell me what had occurred in her life that day. As she began to tell me of her day, she mentioned an incident that occurred earlier on a bus. Someone was mistreating someone else and Lee felt very bad for the person being mistreated. She had not thought much about it after leaving the bus, but upon reaching home, she binged on the waffles and vomited. I asked if perhaps the binging episode and the incident on the bus might be related. She thought a minute and then said, "Yes, I think I identified with the victim. Is that possible?" I told her it certainly was a possibility, but we'd find out more when she came to the session. She then told me that a week earlier she had binged on three bags of carrots. I told her that together we would find out what the behavior means, that there was a reason for the binging, and that it protects her in some way. She hung up seemingly satisfied.

She lived a great distance from my office and had to travel by car to get there. On the morning of her appointment, it snowed heavily. I expected her to cancel the session. To my surprise, she showed up on time and ready to work. It was in this very first session that she told me that she had originally gone to see a psychiatrist and told him of the three pounds of carrots. His response was that this behavior had to stop, and to effect that he would put her on the latest medication that worked in stopping binging. She never went back. She experienced his telling her to stop and his prescription for medication as very controlling. She did not want to be controlled; she had had enough of that in her life. She wanted to be able to feel the control she needed from within herself.

In the following weeks, the therapy was increased to two times per week. Each time there was a binge, we spoke of the necessity of accepting the fact of the binge and explored what occurred in her life the day of or prior to the binging. Slowly, she began to discover that binging and purging were hiding feelings that she did not want to have. She started to realize that her mother and grandmother were constantly interfering in her life. She could not make any choices about anything without them saying something about the choice. She began to realize that her life was not her own, that she lived only to please others and worried constantly about what others thought of her. She did not want to know of her annoyance and anger at the people closest to her, as nice people don't get angry, especially with their relatives. She had been taught this from childhood. She did not think much of herself. She found it especially difficult to care for her two children, as she had so many unmet needs of her own. She wanted no more children ever again—they were just a burden.

Her parents, grandparents, aunts, and uncles were holocaust survivors. Lee was always told that she was lucky to be living in America so that she would not have to be persecuted by the Nazis, that she should appreciate the easy life she had here. Her mother constantly worried that someone would come and take her children from her. She taught the children that the home was the safest place to be, the outside world dangerous. In addition, mother would placate everyone; she never wanted anyone angry with her. Lee and her father fought constantly, and her brothers were often hit by him. He had a very short temper and everyone in the family was careful not to upset him when he was home. In addition, he had a heart condition and mother would warn the children not to upset father as they could cause him to have a heart attack. Thus any assertive feelings or expressions of difference had to be squelched, or father would become upset, could even have a heart attack. Mother, too, would become upset.

The family tolerated no differences among its members. While Lee states that she was her father's favorite, despite her fights with him, he gave the shares in his business to her brothers. She was expected to find a husband to take care of her. When her father died, she was 18; her brothers came into the business as co-owners; she received a small income from the business, but had no say in its operation. She did not realize, until treatment, how bad this made her feel—how insignificant, how stupid, and how upset she was with her dead father. Instead, she had a great deal of guilt concerning her treatment of her father.

In treatment she became aware that her parents' impotent rage against the Nazis had been turned against their children. The victims had become victimizers. The children were the new victims. Mother's fears of being taken prisoner had transferred to her children. Lee also feared that somehow her children would be taken from her. While taught that the safest place to be was at home, Lee felt that she was a prisoner with no life of her own. She felt that somehow she could never make up to her parents for what had been done to them, except by always doing what they asked, never being different from them, never getting angry or upset with them. Yet, she was able to argue with her father, but never with her mother. Moreover, her mother had let her know early on that she was an unwanted and unplanned child.

Each of my patients discussed in this paper never felt accepted by or acceptable to her mother. Hannah and Lee felt some acceptance by their fathers, provided they remained in the subordinate, prescribed role of daddy's little girl. Ann never felt at all accepted by her father, and only acceptable to her mother if she behaved exactly as her mother wanted.

As Lee began to recognize that the binging occurred on days when she was hurt, angry, or upset, she began to feel more in control of her life. It took a year for the binging to stop, and for about a year after that there would be times she would report a binge. My response was always the same: "Well, for some reason you needed to do it. What happened in your life yesterday or the day before?"

After about a year and a half in treatment, Lee, who had been unable to say "no" to anyone, so great was her need to please and to be accepted, began to request changes in her appointment times. Whenever I could, I would change the hour to suit her. I never explored her reasons for the change. Eventually, she questioned her need to do this and decided that it was a way of feeling in control of her own hour as well as a way to say "no" to me. She was, in effect, saying, "No, Eleanor, the hour given me is not suitable. Let's see if I can find one that is more suitable." She also began to question my authority. Working from a self framework, I accepted her questioning as a healthy step in structuralization and validated her right to question the things I say, to challenge me. I agreed that there was no need to accept uncritically all that I said. There were times when she became angry, believing I had misperceived her and what I had said was hurtful to her. Because I believe in accepting the patient's experience of me as she perceives it, I validated her right to be angry with my responses to her without making a transference interpretation. What I found usually happens with all my patients when I validate their experience of me is that they, almost immediately, provide the genetic material.

Because Lee was able to confront me and have her experiences and feelings validated, she began to confront the others in her life. She also began to listen differently to her children to validate their feelings and experiences. At first her mother was hurt by these confrontations, and her response was one guaranteed to provoke guilt. Lee did not suffer her usual guilt feelings, however. Gradually, her mother stopped attacking when confronted and tried to listen to Lee. Although she really could not understand why Lee felt the way she did or experience life the way she did, mother tried to accept Lee's feelings and experiences. Their relationship improved somewhat. Lee was also able to convince her husband to go into therapy.

More and more she began to feel in charge of her life. A happy day occurred when she came to a session and showed me her new shoes. "Do you like them?" she asked. Before I could respond, she said, "Well, it doesn't matter whether you do or don't because I love them." For Lee this was tremendous growth.

After four years of treatment, two of which were totally binge-free, Lee terminated therapy, and she and her husband decided to move to another area. I hear from her from time to time. She had not resumed treatment and has not binged. In a recent letter, she reports that she is pregnant with her third child and writes:

> I'm in the beginning of my 6th month and have put on about 10 pounds since the beginning of my pregnancy . . . when I was pregnant with [my first and second] I started weighing more than I do now. I have started to feel the baby move, and it is very exciting for me. I am enjoying my pregnancy at this point, and am pretty content.

Conclusion

The bulimic patient has not received adequate empathic mirroring. Nor have adequate idealization and deidealization processes taken place, leaving deficits in the self-structure. The patient tries to compensate for these by binging and purging.

Our function as therapists is to provide adequate empathic mirroring, provide an atmosphere in which idealization and deidealization can take place, and help the patient believe in the validity of her own subjective experiences (Stolorow et al., 1987, p. 133). When we do this, transmuting internalizations take place, building self-structure and repairing the deficits in the self. Self-cohesion begins. This allows for the beginnings of self-soothing, self-regulation, self-esteem, and frustration tolerance. The episodes of binging and purging will lessen, and the patient can begin to work with painful material and allow herself to be in touch with painful affects. As the self continues to grow stronger, the patient more and more develops the inner resources to cope with life's vicissitudes. Binging and purging are no longer needed.

References

Bandchaft, B., & Stolorow, R. D. (1984). A current perspective on difficult patients. In P. Stepansky & A. Goldberg (Eds.), *Kohut's legacy: Contributions to self psychology.* Hillsdale, NJ: Analytic Press.

Barth, D. & Wurman, V. (1986). Group therapy with bulimic women: A self-psychological approach. *International Journal of Eating Disorders, 5,* 735–745.

Bemis, K. M. (1985). "Abstinence" and "non-abstinence" models for the treatment of bulimia. *International Journal of Eating Disorders, 4,* 407–437.

Bruch, H. (1973). *Eating disorders: Obesity, anorexia nervosa and the person within.* New York: Basic Books.
Cauwels, J. (1983). *Bulimia: The binge-purge compulsion.* New York: Doubleday.
Goodsit, A. (1983). Self-regulatory disturbances in eating disorders. *International Journal of Eating Disorders, 2,* 51–60.
Greenson, R. (1978). The real relationship between the patient and the psychoanalyst. In *Explorations in psychoanalysis.* New York: International Universities Press.
Kohut, H. (1971). *The analysis of the self.* New York: International Universities Press.
Kohut, H. (1977). *The restoration of the self.* New York: International Universities Press.
Magid, B. (1984). Some contributions of self psychology to the treatment of borderline and schizophrenic patients. *Dynamic Psychotherapy, 2,* 101–111.
Neuman, P., & Halvorson, P. (1983). *Anorexia nervosa and bulimia: A handbook for counselors and therapists.* New York: Van Nostrand Reinhold.
Stolorow, R., Bandchaft, B., & Atwood, G. (1987). *Psychoanalytic treatment: An intersubjective approach.* Hillsdale, NJ: Analytic Press.
Stepansky, P., & Goldberg, A. (1984). *Kohut's legacy: Contributions to self psychology.* Hillsdale, NJ: Analytic Press.
Sugarman, A., & Kurash, C. (1982). The body as a transitional object in bulimia. *International Journal of Eating Disorders, 1,* 44–61.
Swift, W. J., & Letven, R. (1984). Bulimia and the basic fault: A psychoanalytic interpretation of the binging-vomiting syndrome. *Journal of the American Academy of Child Psychiatry, 23*(4), 489–497.
Tolpin, M. (1971). On the beginning of a cohesive self: An application of the concept of transmuting internalization to the study of transitional objects and anxiety. *Psychoanalytic Study of the Child, 26,* 316–352.
Welbourne, J., & Purgold, J. (1984). *The eating sickness: Anorexia, bulimia and the myth of suicide by slimming.* Brighton, Sussex: Harvester Press.